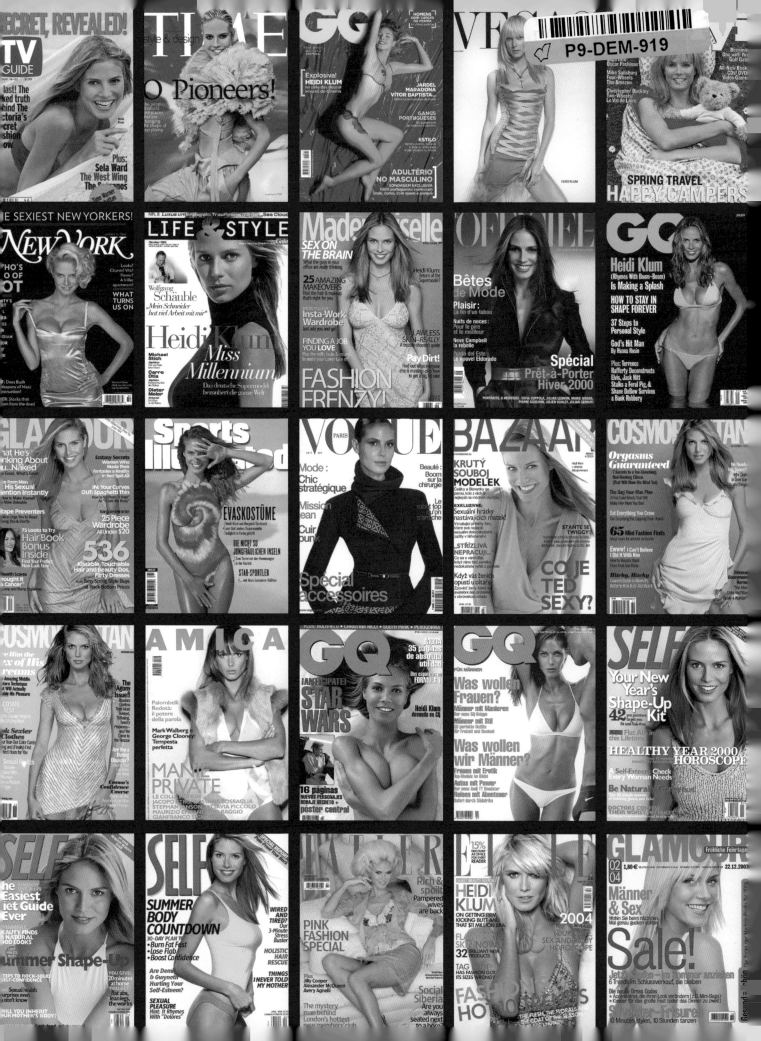

# HEIDI KLUM'S
## body of knowledge

**8
RULES OF
MODEL BEHAVIOR**
(to Help You Take Off
on the Runway of Life)

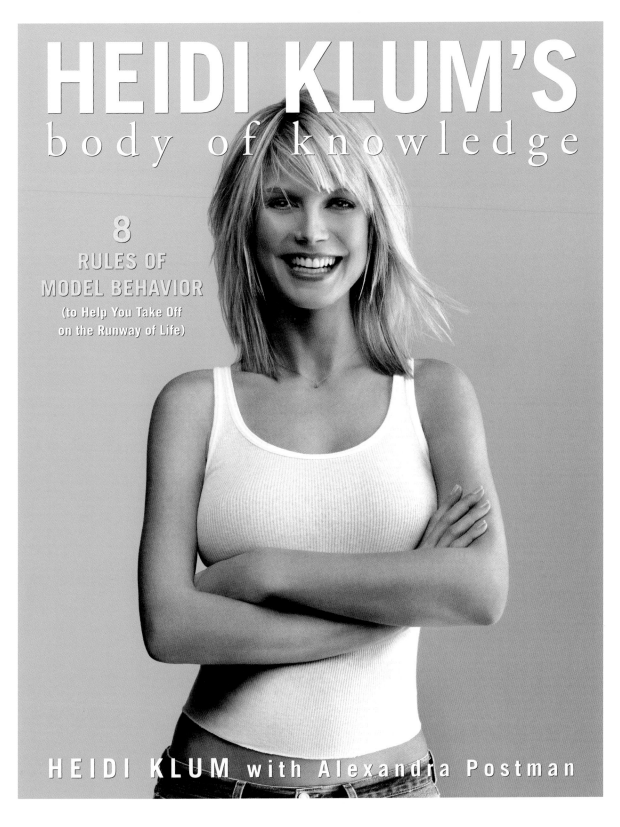

## HEIDI KLUM with Alexandra Postman

CROWN PUBLISHERS / NEW YORK

Published by Crown Publishers, New York, New York

Member of the Crown Publishing Group, a division of Random House, Inc.

www.crownpublishing.com

CROWN is a trademark and the Crown colophon is a registered trademark of Random House, Inc.

Printed in the United States of America

Design by Elizabeth Van Itallie

Library of Congress Cataloging-in-Publication Data

Klum, Heidi.

      Heidi Klum's body of knowledge : 8 rules of model behavior (to help you take off on the runway of life) / Heidi Klum with Alexandra Postman.

          p.  cm.

      1. Models (Persons)—Vocational guidance.  2. Models (Persons)—Conduct of life.

3. Models (Persons)—Biography.  I. Title: Body of Knowledge : 8 rules of model behavior (to help you take off on the runway of life).  II. Postman, Alexandra S., 1968–  III. Title.

      HD8039.M77K58 2004

      650.1—dc22                                      2004000070

ISBN 1-4000-5028-6

10  9  8  7  6  5  4  3  2  1

First Edition

I want to thank my team—
you all know who you are—and the people
who gave me a chance.

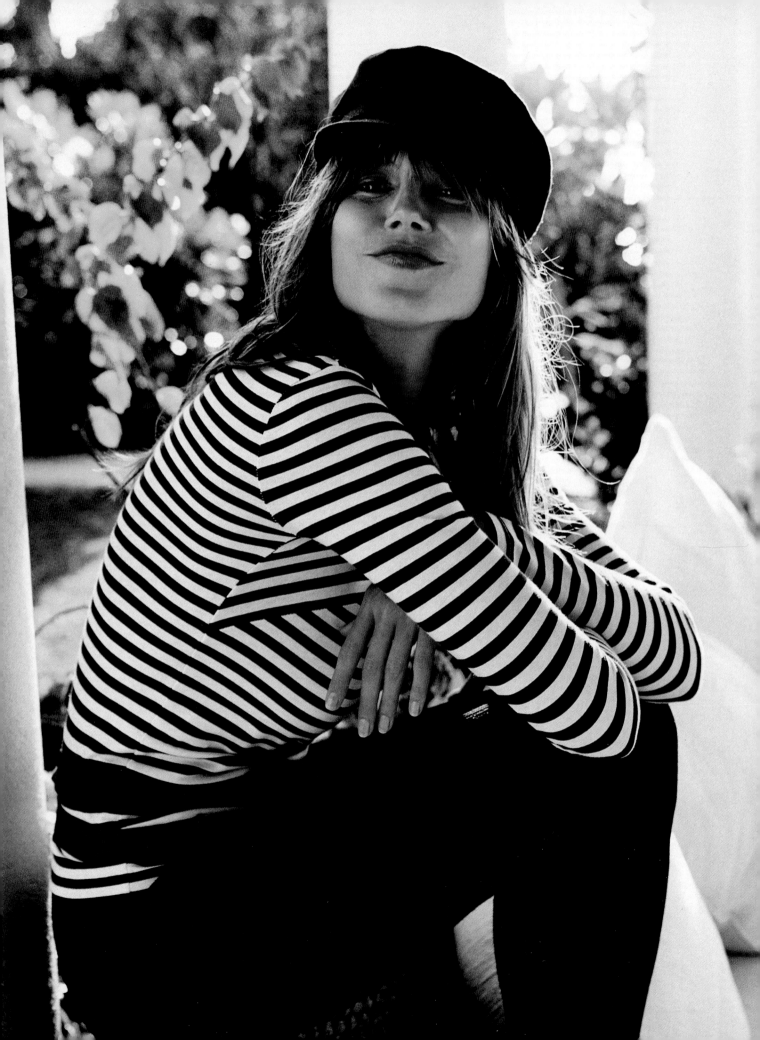

# contents

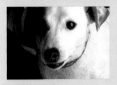

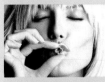

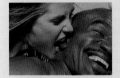

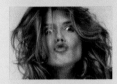

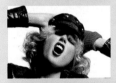

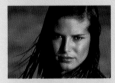

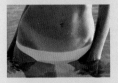

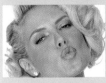

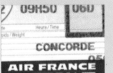

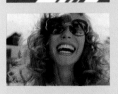

# introduction

Yeah, yeah. I know.

Where does a model—okay, *super*model—get off telling you how to look your absolute best, or how to attract the opposite sex, or anything except maybe how to wear a pair of pants so your butt looks great or how to put just the right amount of hip action into a turn at the end of the runway? Who the hell am I? What does a globe-trotting, supposedly pampered cover girl know about the struggle to look good (or just good enough), to make one's hair, skin, and abs all that they can be, or to find Mr. Right?

Fair questions. Now I'd like to answer them.

First, whatever you may think about what models do (pose, drink, smoke, catfight, look bored, have lots of sex), it's not just about looking pretty (or pouty) for a lensman. Second, because so many people think what we do *is* just about looking pretty, it's unbelievably competitive. And third, succeeding in such a competitive business—as in *any* competitive business—requires two equal, sometimes opposite, abilities:

The ability to play the game and the ability to beat the game.

But when I say "the game," I don't just mean the game of modeling. I mean the game of Life.

The thing is, as I've become a better-known (and, I hope, just plain better) model, there are several "rules" of the trade I've mastered. Some of them I've picked up from watching those with more experience; some of them are self-taught. Taken together, these rules make up my own book of "Model Behavior"—stuff that successful models learn, understand, and use (and, granted, sometimes exploit). At some point it occurred to me that if knowing and following these rules can help someone communicate so well with a mere camera (and thrive as a model), then maybe they could also help *you* communicate well with the rest of the world (and thrive as a person). Certainly these rules—or principles to live by, if you like—have done that for me and rewarded me with a life I could never have had otherwise.

But maybe I still haven't answered your question. Why me?

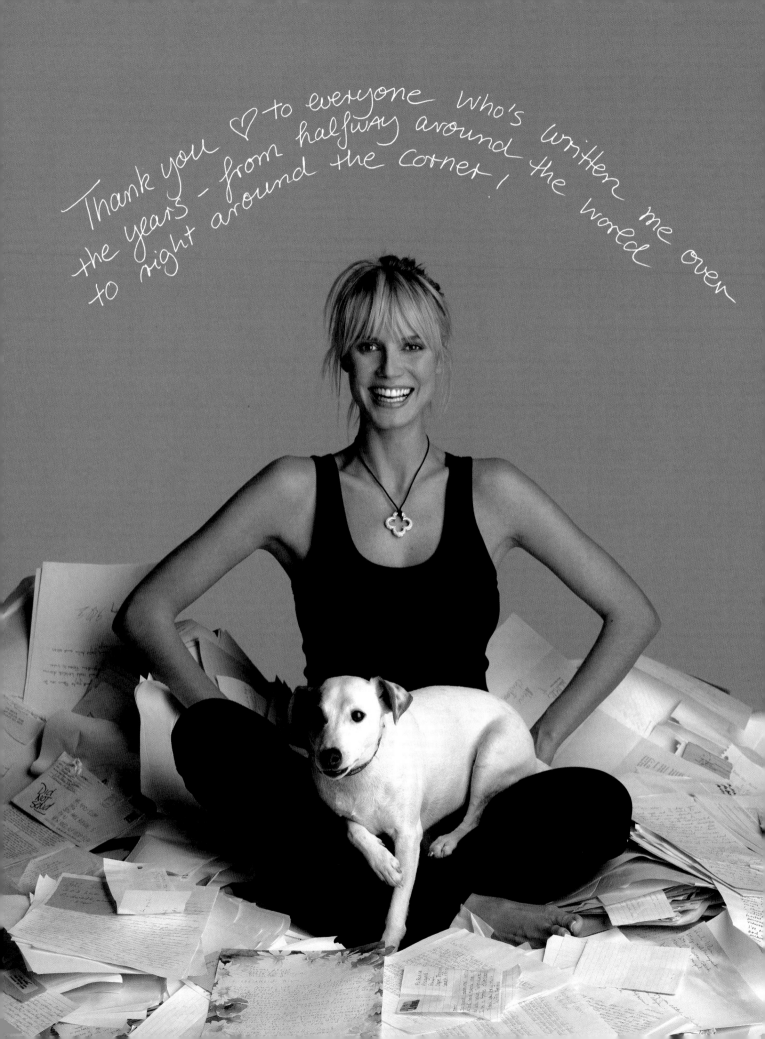

Thank you ♡ to everyone who's written me over the years – from halfway around the world to right around the corner!

A former small-town girl, I never expected to make it as far as I have. But the fact that I have created this life (modeling contracts, my own calendar, clothing and jewelry lines, TV and movie gigs) qualifies me, I think, to talk about how to get the most out of oneself. That sounds arrogant, right? But I think it's exactly the opposite. Because I'm no better-looking than lots and lots—and *lots*—of models out there. Want the truth? I'm shorter than most of them, and heavier, plus I smile a lot. Not exactly a stock in trade. I have what I call a German butt, probably from eating too many potatoes.

So why'd *I* graduate to the next level?

Sure, I have some natural assets (make the obvious jokes), but if I hadn't pushed every agent I've worked with to help me get more challenging, high-profile modeling work; and created opportunities by keeping an open mind and exploring new ventures; and urged every producer to beef up my role; and gone out of my way to actually be nice to people I meet because—who knows?—you just might learn something from them (and, quite frankly, why not?), I wouldn't have made it beyond my first catalog job.

> You make your own bed. So you might as well sleep on a king-size mattress with silk sheets.

Everyone has strengths. But not everyone experiences as much success and enjoyment from life as they'd like, or are entitled to. To quote Julia Roberts's enthusiastic Oscar speech, *I love my life.* I know I've had a lot of success. But it didn't happen by accident. In my opinion, a lot of the pleasure we experience, maybe most, comes from how we feel about ourselves, how we carry ourselves, and what we can make other people think we're capable of. Even a fashion model (maybe *especially* a fashion model) could have a few worthwhile things to say on those subjects.

Reason number two that qualifies me to write this book: my jet-setty lifestyle. What I mean is that my work has granted me access to famous, successful people who love talking about how they got that way. (In fact, some of them have done me the honor of letting me print their advice in these pages.) And since I've spent great chunks of time flying from New York to Milan to Bali to Japan to If-It's-Tuesday-This-Must-Be-Cancún (the boarding passes shown in this book are from the planet's largest collection—mine), I've also had loads of time to strategize about what I want from life, and how to make it happen.

Oh, yeah, and a *third* reason: We supermodels are famous for getting our way.

So I hope you'll pick up a tip or five here, be inspired to try something new or get creative with your own life, look at some of my favorite pictures by the photographers I most admire (including Mom and Dad), and maybe have a few laughs at my expense. Not that I mind! Humility is actually a big part of building resilience and success.

I mean, I pig out, work out, and get pimples like everyone else. In fact, thanks to my adolescent acne, some snotty kids in high school used to call me Pizza Face. Still, I'm not going to pretend I lived some kind of ugly-duckling story—you know, Gawky Teen Spotted in Airport Lands on Cover of Major Magazine. I was late to develop, but I did have a couple of boyfriends and a pretty normal social life.

Now that you know my teenage nickname, I'd like to take a moment to clear up some other misinformation that's been generated about me. It's funny how something that you do or say to a reporter can get taken out of context and then follow you around forever. Next thing you know, you do an interview and the reporter asks:

**Heidi, do you really yodel after sex?**

No! That was just something the producers of the American sitcom *Spin City* developed for my character (I played Michael J. Fox's love interest for six episodes). We don't yodel where I come from in Germany—that's more of a Bavarian thing. But somehow people have this idea that all German women wear pigtails and dirndls and keep a cuckoo clock on the wall. I've vacationed in the Alps since I was a child and picked up a little yodeling, which I've demonstrated a few times in TV interviews. But I promise you I've never belted out a post-coital yodel.

**I've read that you carry your baby teeth with you when you travel. True?**

You got me there. First of all, you should know that I collect and keep everything. Old love letters, art projects, even my teeth. I have all my baby teeth; I even have my wisdom teeth. I store them in a little leather pouch that I found on a trip to Phoenix, and at some point I started traveling with it. If I don't have my teeth with me I worry the plane's going to crash or something. It started as a superstition but now it's a pain, because I always have to lug them around the world with me.

**What's up with those crazy Halloween costumes?**

I love a good theme party, and I start planning my annual Halloween bash in July. In previous years, I've been everything from Lady Godiva, Betty Boop, and a space alien to "Hard-Core Heidi." Not the most glamorous costumes, perhaps, but all incredibly fun to put together. What I love best about these parties is watching all of my guests try to figure out who's who: Hey, is that P. Diddy dressed as King Louis XIV?

**One last question. Are those real?**

Okay, the boobs? Can't get around those. Funny how much attention they get, huh? A reporter once asked me what message I was trying to send with my breasts. Message? I asked. They have no message. They just have to fit in the bra.

Once and for all, they *are* real—100 percent as nature made them.

So I guess we've come full circle: Maybe I have something worthwhile to say because the Rules of Model Behavior, which I've long followed, are all about making the most out of what I have.

Why can't they benefit you, too, and help you to satisfy what you need and want?

In fact, before we start, do yourself one favor: Imagine a compliment you'd love to be paid, in the near future—by a stranger, a friend, your landlord, doesn't matter. Something they totally mean and can't help saying. And I'm not referring to the usual clichés of "nice hair" or "great shoes." Some of the best compliments are roundabout—testaments to your persistence, loyalty, or some other character strength. To get you started, here are a few of my favorites:

## 10 COMPLIMENTS YOU'D LOVE TO EARN

1. "Boy, you don't take no for an answer, do you?"
2. "How'd you pull *that* off?"
3. "You're glowing!" (Doesn't count if you're pregnant. Or drunk.)
4. "I'd be honored to be your wingman."
5. "Who does your wardrobe?" (Especially if the answer is *you*.)
6. "I could learn a lot from you."
7. "You're a human Energizer bunny."
8. "You handled that situation nicely."
9. "When did you have time to do all that?"
10. "Great ass!" (double points if from the same sex)

Now, let's figure out how to win that kind of praise.

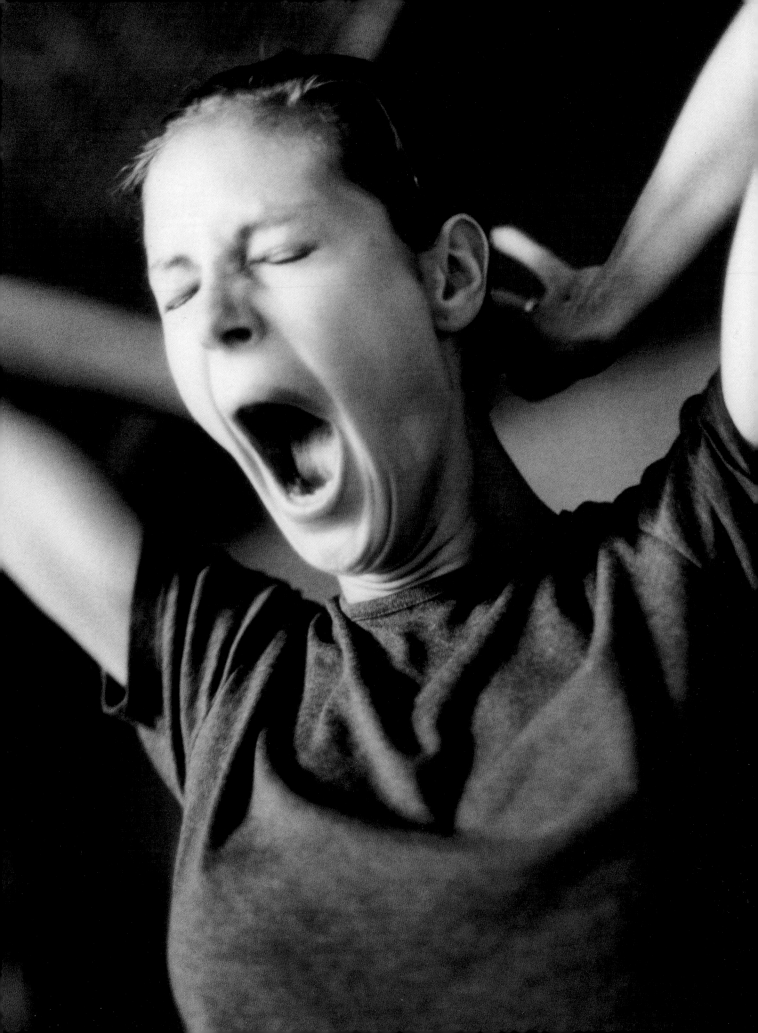

# DESIRE

**RULE 1**

*you have to*
## want it, baby

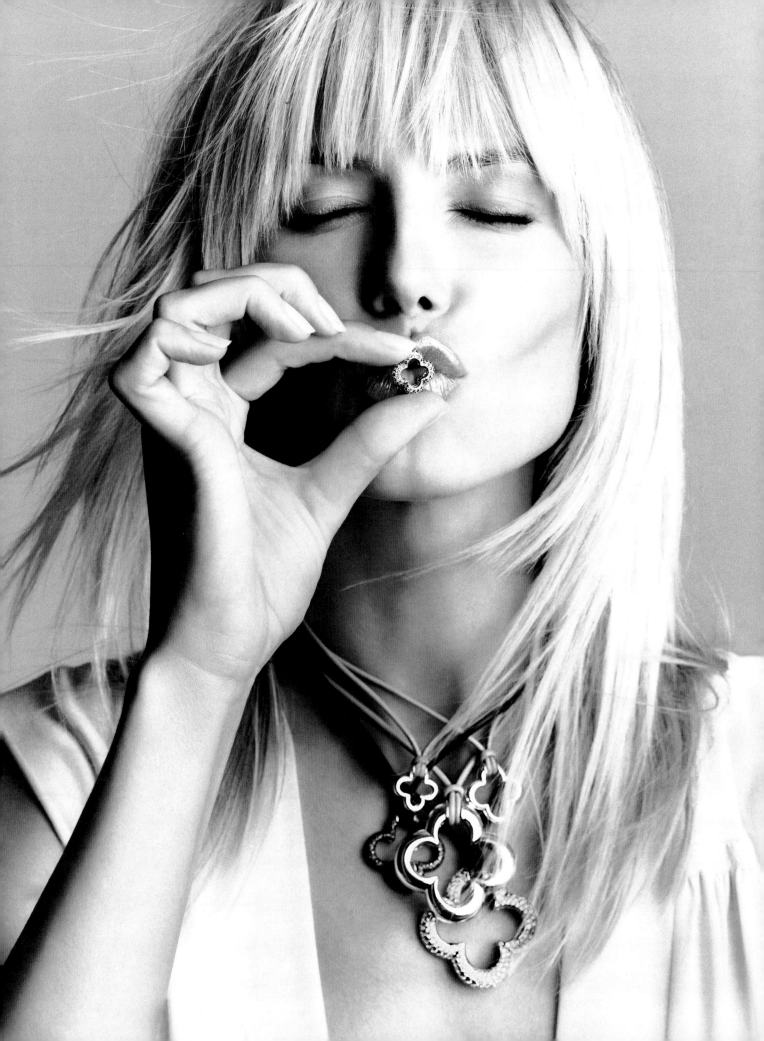

**M**odeling is about desire. Oh, sure, it's about other things, too—beauty, selling clothes, presenting an artistic vision. But when the camera snaps, it's not enough for us models just to stand there looking pretty or sexy. The bottom line is that we have to present ourselves in such a way that the viewer wants us, wants to be like us, or at least wants what we're wearing . . . or sipping . . . or driving. We have to spark desire, make you feel it in a powerful way.

And how do we do that? Easy.

*We* have to want it.

I was one of those who really, *really* wanted it.

Wanted what? Not to be famous, but to get to the top of my field and lead the fullest life I knew how.

Does it suck to show up at a casting call and find hundreds of girls lined up, all over five foot ten, all gorgeous, all trying to get the job that you covet? Yes, it does, if you were me, a recent arrival to New York, wanting badly to become a model and not knowing when or if it would happen. (No, it doesn't suck if you're some guy standing on the sidewalk, using every line in the book to hit on three hundred girls.)

Luckily, though, I had one thing going for me besides a better-than-average face and body: I wanted it bad. Don't get me wrong: Hard work is key. Ability is key. A degree of luck is key. But desire is the ultimate motivator. It makes you work like crazy and not give up too fast or too easily. The thing you always hear about Michael Jordan is that he was the greatest basketball player not because he was the most talented (though he was), but because he was the most driven and compet-itive—all the time. Same with Tiger Woods. But this is true not just of super-stars but also of most everyone who has done incredibly well in their profession. They just want it more.

Do you want to make a better life? Do you?

Through the power of wanting, you make life happen, rather than sitting back and waiting for opportunities to find you (ain't gonna happen), or relying on others to make things happen for you. I know it's a cliché to say *If you see it, you can be it.* But I totally believe that: You can't get what you want if you don't express it. So I say: Ask for it. Ask yourself, ask your parents, your friends, your boss, your boss's boss, your agent, your respective deity.

Here are a few of my earliest modeling assign-ments (check out my first nude shoot in Italy, and that sassy hand-on-hip pose that's stuck with me all these years). I've never shied away from the sound of the camera snapping!

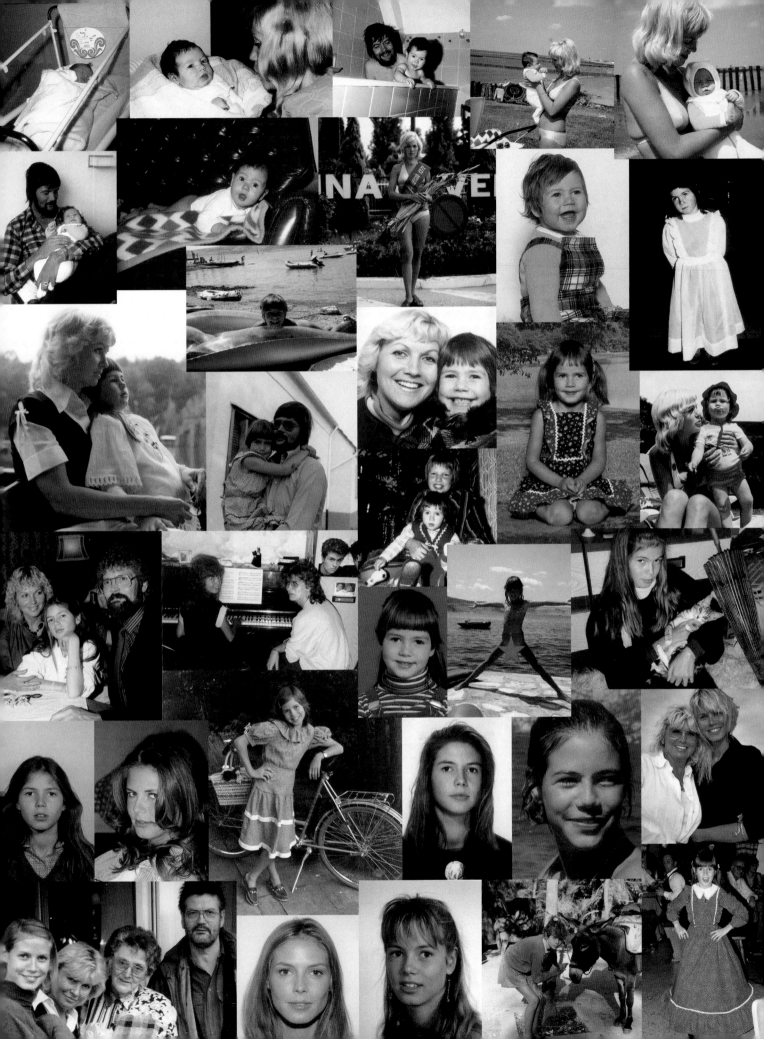

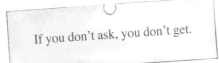

Now you know my personal motto.

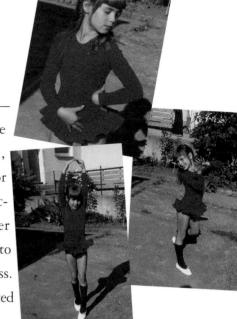

## attitude creates opportunity

I never could have predicted the path my life has taken—but from the time I was a little girl growing up in the small town of Bergisch-Gladbach near Cologne, Germany, I was raised to have high expectations for myself. My dad, Günther, a cosmetics executive, was strict with me and my older brother, Michael, but he encouraged me to be opinionated, self-assured, and fearless. My mom, Erna, a hairstylist, is big-hearted and down-to-earth; she taught me empathy and optimism, to prize my freedom, and to never have to depend on a man. So from my earliest years, I was ambitious and motivated (not that I had everything figured out by the time I was ten).

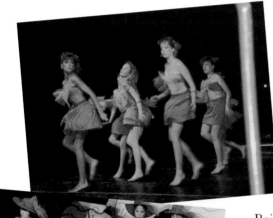

Being raised in a very loving, nurturing family also gave me a sense of confidence and an emotional safety net. We spent a lot of time together—we'd sit around the dinner table talking about our days at work and school, our vacation plans, our friends. In hindsight, I was fortunate to have known that I was loved and protected, as well as to have learned the importance of manners, of common courtesy and mutual respect. From that feeling of security in my family life, I grew up confident enough to try different paths in life without being scared or intimidated all the time.

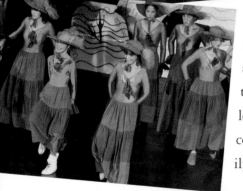

I was always a ham; I loved being onstage—I started ballet at age five and always felt natural in front of a big crowd. I took tap, jazz, ballet, even belly-dancing and ballroom for many years, until I left for New York at age nineteen. Throughout high school, I performed with my local dance troupe—it wasn't Broadway but for my town it was a big deal—and traveled the country to compete. I may not have been the best student academically, but in dance I found something that I loved, excelled at, and was passionate about.

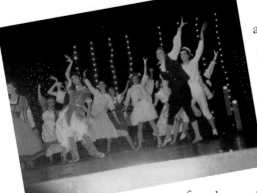

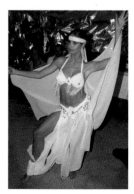

As part of a team, I felt the gratification of contributing to a larger effort, but watching the best dancers in the first row of class also got my competitive juices flowing, because even back then, I wanted to be good. So from an early age I knew that ambition and goal-setting are important . . . and fun.

When I wasn't actually onstage, I'd sometimes pretend to be. My best friend Karin and I were huge Wham! fans. She loved George Michael and I was into Andrew Ridgeley. (I loved his puppy eyes.) So Karin and I would use a tape recorder and a one-meter-long Schnapps bottle for a microphone, and we'd tape ourselves singing out loud. At night, when it got dark outside, the windows would become huge mirrors and we'd be dancing and singing to the music.

So I guess you could say that performing and being "on" have always been natural and fun for me. At the time, though, I had no concept of the modeling world. I knew about Claudia Schiffer because she was German, but I didn't aspire to be like her or anything. I came from a little town. Who the hell would find me there?

One day when we were eighteen, Karin and I were flipping through magazines when she showed me a promotion for a modeling contest that had been airing for weeks on TV—hosted by Thomas Gottschalk, Germany's biggest talk-show emcee—in which the weekly winners competed for a prize. "They're still looking for girls,"

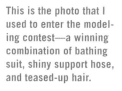

This is the photo that I used to enter the modeling contest—a winning combination of bathing suit, shiny support hose, and teased-up hair.

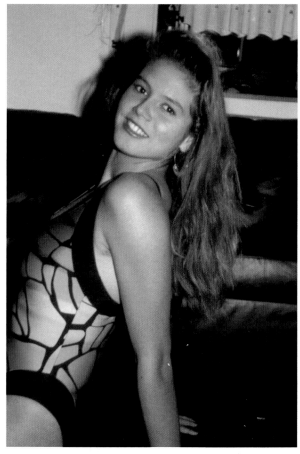

Karin said. "You should try it!" We watched the show that week. Karin and I couldn't stop laughing at how silly the girls looked sitting there, dumbfounded. We just trashed the whole thing. But Karin urged me to enter.

On a lark, I put on my shiny tight dance stockings and a bathing suit (a fashion no-no!), teased up my hair, and smeared on a lot of blush. We took Polaroids, filled out the coupon, and sent it all in. After nearly five months I still hadn't heard anything (and had pretty much forgotten about the whole thing). Out of the blue, I got a phone call from one of the show's representatives inviting me to Munich for a casting call. I didn't even know what that meant! My parents were away on a trip, and I was too scared to go alone (and too excited not to go), so I called my ex-boyfriend to drive me down. Six hours later, I was sitting in a huge room packed with girls around my age, from whom they were going to pick contestants. When my name was called, I went into a back room where the casting team interrogated me about my hobbies, my schoolwork, etc. Then they thanked me and sent me off saying, "Don't call us, we'll call you."

The very next day, they did. I'd made the final cut. I couldn't believe it. I'd entered this thing on a dare, and next thing I knew I was going to appear on national television.

Two weeks later, my mom, who was as giddy as I was, drove me back to Munich to tape my clip. (My father, ever the realist, warned me not to get my hopes up.) In the video, each girl had to dance in front of a mirror to a song—mine was "Music Was My First Love"—and then stand under a fake waterfall while water cascaded over us (we also had to lie on an air mattress that was floating on a pool, and paddle past the camera for a close-up). I found the whole thing a bit ridiculous, and thought I sounded as silly as the girls Karin and I had mocked. That's what happens when you're nervous as hell. But when the audience called in and voted . . . I won!

After another round against that month's winners, I qualified for the finals. At this point I was something of a local celebrity, because everyone watched the show. I was getting teased in school and the other girls, probably out of jealousy, started whispering about me behind my back. (That's when I started building up a protective shell against scrutiny and criticism.) When I returned to Munich for the last round, even my skeptical father came along. The whole way there he alternated between preparing me for the worst, and warning me against getting a big head.

Personally, I didn't think I stood a chance. I was up against five other girls, all of whom seemed pretty and talented. The producers put us all—wearing our big dresses and teased hair—in the backseat of a convertible, and we rode onto the stage, where we had to do a cooking segment frying dough balls while answering questions about ourselves. Next we did a fashion show. The audience voted to eliminate three out of the six, and those of us remaining were evaluated by a panel of five judges. And then it was time. The announcer walked to the mike seemingly in slow motion. We were huddled behind the door when we heard him say, "And the winner of Model '92 is . . . Heidi Klum!"

The spotlight caught me in its glare while fireworks showered down, and the entire audience stood on their feet, cheering. Out of 30,000 girls, I was the winner. Thomas Gottschalk passed me a bouquet of exotic flowers. The whole thing was like a weird dream—most of all when, after the show, a representative from the sponsoring modeling agency handed me a piece of paper awarding me a three-year contract for a purported $300,000.

My father grabbed the document and gave it a quick read. Then he folded it up

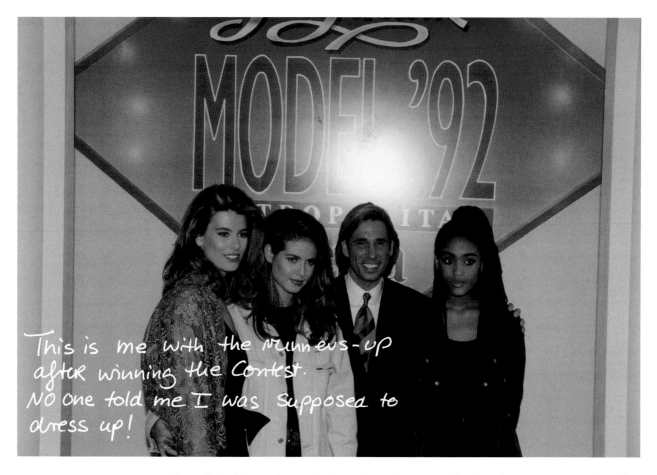

*This is me with the runners-up after winning the Contest. NO One told me I was supposed to dress up!*

and put it in his pocket. "Yeah, we're going to need a few days to go over that," he said. The agency rep looked stunned, and started to protest. "We have to show this to a lawyer," my father said. "There's a lot of language in there that I don't understand, and certainly my daughter doesn't understand it."

It turned out my father was right.

## down and out in milan and paris

Overnight, I'd become a nationally recognizable figure—I was on TV and my picture was in all the newspapers. The attention was a little overwhelming, and even more unbelievable. I figured I'd do a bit of modeling here and there while living at home, then go back to school to become a clothing designer. Meantime, however, despite the accolades, the modeling jobs weren't exactly falling in my lap. My father's lawyers had found a loophole in the contract saying the agency wasn't obligated to pay me the award unless I found enough work—fortunately we fought it, and they ended up guaranteeing me the money. But since they were paying me no matter what, they didn't exactly hustle to find me jobs.

This opportunity had landed in my lap and I was determined to make a go of my new career. At the start, I had no book, no pictures, nothing. Still, they sent me to Paris and Milan to meet with photographers, but it didn't really lead to much. In Germany, it was a little easier to get work. I got a spread in *Freundin* magazine and other small German publications. I also landed in more than one knitting magazine. It certainly wasn't *Vogue*—but it was a start.

My first really beautiful pictures appeared in *Petra*, a popular women's magazine (the same one where I'd found the coupon for the contest). They came to my house (it was during one of my phases where everything in my room was green, from the walls to the AstroTurf floor) and put me in this gorgeous cotton-candy–colored Chanel dress with cascading glass Chanel earrings and accessories, and styled my hair and makeup so I looked like a movie star. I remember the first time I saw the spread in the magazine, I barely recognized myself.

In Paris, I went to hundreds of castings and got only a handful of jobs. I did some lingerie modeling for a no-name Italian company. I did a TV spot for the Swatch

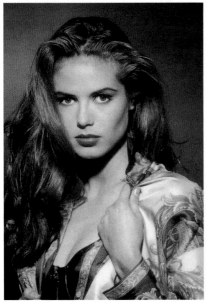

**BELOW:** My first autograph card—for all 10 of my fans. **OPPOSITE:** My first published photos ran in *Petra*. Fake lashes . . . Chanel couture . . . flashy jewelry . . . Bring it on!

phone. Back then, the whole Kate Moss waif look was in—all sunken cheekbones and stuck-out ribs—and I was told over and over again that my looks were too normal, too girl-next-door, too American pie. I had big boobs and curvy hips, which were out of fashion in the early 1990s. In Milan, where I traveled every so often, the agency started coaching me on my appearance—I needed tighter clothes, higher heels, not too much makeup, simple hair. And, oh, yeah, there was that special "mix": "Mix this with that and drink it so you'll lose weight," they urged. They also stripped me down and weighed and measured me, keeping rigorous records. I felt like a piece of meat. I wasn't going to drink that water, and I refused to show up at parties populated with guys who expected me to sleep with them. I was straight as a button.

It was around this time that I decided to go to America.

# if you can make it there, you'll make it anywhere

I called up the modeling agency's main office in New York and asked if I could come there to work. The agency told me to stop off in Miami first for test pictures.

I flew to Miami in October of 1993. I was nineteen years old, and I tried a little too hard to stand out: I wore crazy clothes like snakeskin cowboy boots and leather vests, and I troweled on the makeup. The agency set me up at a cheap hotel filled with other models, and within days, someone broke into my room and stole my passport and credit cards. I went on casting after casting—I'd arrive in some hotel

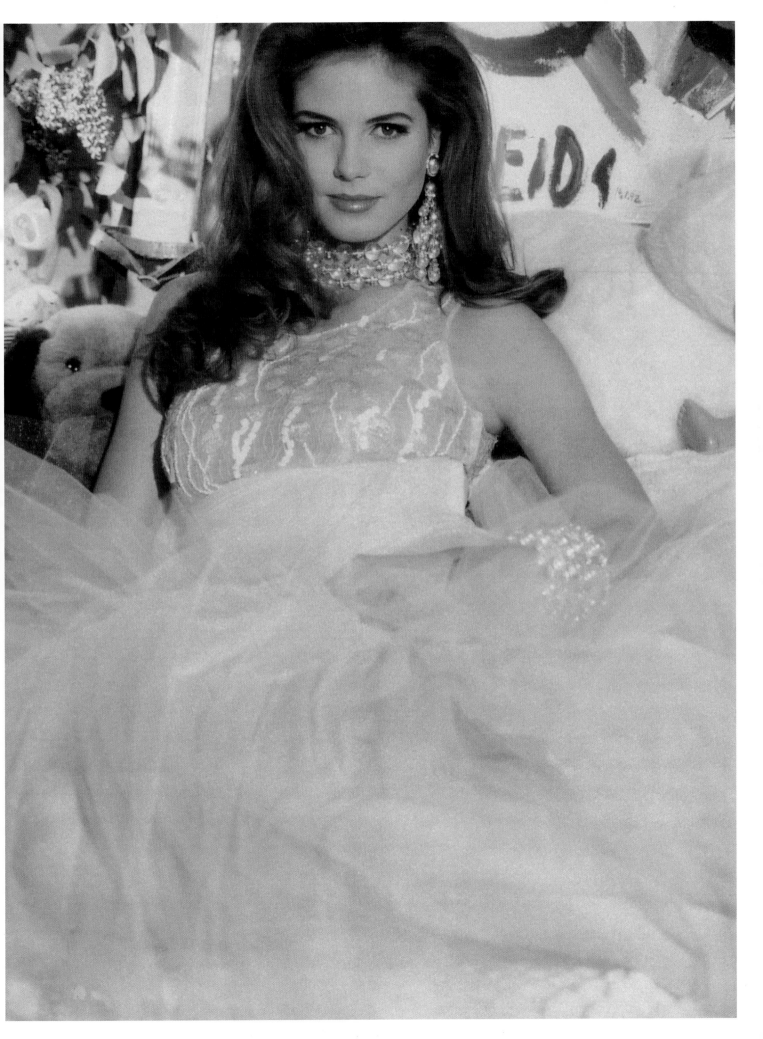

lobby that would be teeming with models, and I'd be number 205. I figured it would be more productive to focus on building up my portfolio, so I paid for more test shots—about $200 a pop. On tests, typically the photographer's girlfriend does your makeup and you wear some clothes out of her closet. But tests are really important because they can demonstrate to a casting agent what you look like in different styles. Plus it gives you a chance to stand in front of a camera.

After a month, I'd had just about enough. If parties are your thing, then Miami is The Place to be. Despite the balmy weather and sandy beaches, Miami is a harsh environment in which to thrive as a model. I knew a lot of starving models who would go out with men just to get a decent meal, but the guys would invariably want more at the end of the day. Me, I wasn't getting anywhere fast. More than ever, I longed to go to New York. I wanted to hit the real fashion capital.

I called my agency in New York and asked if I could come. Actually, I pretty much told them I was coming. I wouldn't take no for an answer.

They sent me a ticket and told me that someone would be at the airport to pick me up. Of course, nobody showed. All I had was a piece of paper with my agent's phone number and the address of where they were putting me up (I'd have to reimburse them the $800 a month rent from my earnings). I didn't even have my winter clothes with me, because I was supposed to be in Miami.

Lucky for me, I met a photographer on the plane and we shared a cab into the city. Driving into Manhattan was so overwhelming, so much to take in at once—the skyscrapers, the lights, the bridges, the people . . . Holy cow! It felt just like a movie.

The taxi dropped me off at my apartment, a dilapidated brownstone on Eighteenth Street between First and Second Avenues. The agency had set me up with two German roommates—in one respect, kind of a bummer because I wanted to learn English, but they instantly made me feel at home. Julia and Bianca filled me in on the dirt (literally): The building had no hot water. There were leaks in the ceiling. The whole place was crawling with cockroaches.

I got my first taste of celebrity right away: Julia happened to be dating Prince. On some nights, he'd come pick her up in a long stretch limo. When she'd go downstairs to meet him, Bianca and I would press our noses against the window to catch a glimpse, but he'd always stay in the car. We knew it was him, though, because he wrote the song "The Most Beautiful Girl in the World" for her, and we heard it two years before it was ever released.

Every single day for three months I went on casting calls, sometimes as many as ten a day. I was just one of thousands of new girls trying to make it as a model in New York, and every one of them looked fabulous. Typically I'd wait in line and the client would look at my book, thank me, and send me packing. It sucked being such a small fish in a big pond.

> If 90 percent of life is just showing up—I just kept showing up.

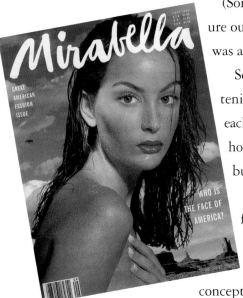

(Sometimes I showed up at the wrong address: It took me several weeks to figure out that Manhattan streets are divided into East and West sides.) Everything was a learning process—a process in learning how to "do it yourself."

Soon, I started having weight problems because I couldn't resist all the fattening American food—the muffins and brownies and candies. At the end of each day, I would sit around with my roommates, and we'd be sourpussing about how little work we were getting. Julia gave up and went back to Germany, but I didn't want to go home just yet. So I swallowed hard and stuck it out.

Then, finally, I got my first big job. Not only was it a job, it was a cover for *Mirabella*, a prestigious fashion magazine, and the photographer was the famous Japanese lensman Hiro. I'd never heard of him. I'd never heard of *any* big-name photographers, for that matter, but it was all good to me. The concept was the "perfect woman." The shoot took hours because Hiro was very particular about my makeup. When I finally glanced in the mirror, it looked as if a sculptor had been working on me: My face was molded with light and shadows to bring out my cheekbones, the mascara was applied perfectly, my eyebrows plucked just right. Hiro put a microchip in my ear for a finishing touch.

A few weeks later, as I was walking down the street thinking that the issue would soon be out, I stopped in my tracks in front of a newsstand. There was *Mirabella* . . . with another girl on the cover. She was even wearing my microchip in her ear! I was so mad. Then I read the story, which explained that Hiro had synthesized the best features from six models to create a composite of the Perfect Woman. At least I had one-sixth of a cover. And a funny story for my book.

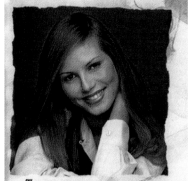

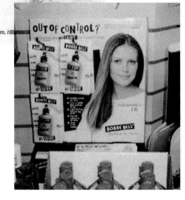

After the Hiro shoot, things started to move a little. I got a job representing the cosmetics line Bonne Bell and saw my face splashed across makeup displays in every drugstore. That was cool. Meanwhile, I was still doing castings. I got a job for *YM* magazine and a cover for *Bride's,* but continued to do lots of test pictures.

My first big break was a stroke of luck. But it shows that if you constantly push yourself and take small steps toward a goal, you'll create opportunities you might not have had otherwise. At this point in my career, I could never have gotten a *real* cover. Big models get covers. If you're lucky, at my level, you got editorial work on the inside.

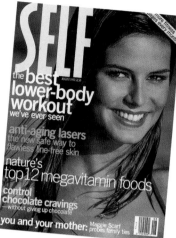

But luck intervened in the form of photographer Michael Zeppetello. He was doing a shoot for *YM* and searching for girls that looked athletic and approachable. He cast me and four other girls and we went to Anguilla. We did the shoot for *YM,* but he also took some test photos while we were down there, in the event that someone would see the final result, like them, and publish them. (Editorial work doesn't earn you as much money as advertising, but it gets your face out there, which just might lead to more work.) We spent two days shooting creative, beautiful pictures—head shots, bathing suit shots, etc. Shortly after we got back, one of those pictures landed on the cover of *Self.* The magazine came out in August 1995. In less than a year in New York, I was poised to break into the big time. But I couldn't have foreseen that it would take me another four years . . .

## the catalog queen

Right before I made the cover of *Self,* I'd signed a year-round contract with Newport News, a women's clothing catalog. I must have been selling a lot of clothes, because I worked constantly for them. We'd shoot in Miami for two weeks, then jet down to Cabo San Lucas for another two. Meantime, I was also doing work for JC Penney and Chadwick's. I was the catalog queen, on the road 220 days of the year—which was exceptionally hard since I'd recently met the man who would soon become my husband (Ric Pipino) and we worked hard at stoking the romantic flames from halfway around the globe.

But I was in a trap. My agency had a good deal; they didn't have to do any hustling on my behalf. I was the horse that was running all over the place making money, and they were getting the commission. So after the third year of my contract from the modeling contest, I left my agency to go to a rival agency, Elite. They hadn't gotten me the Newport News contract, but they were already raking in the money from all my clients. And it wasn't insubstantial: In the beginning, I would get $1,500 a day. Then it was $5,000 a day, and eventually it was $10,000. I bought a house for everyone in my family—my brother, my aunt, my parents. But catalog work just wasn't very fulfilling or challenging. I wanted to see if I could get to the next level.

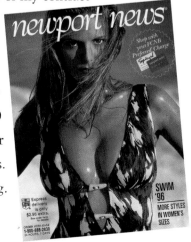

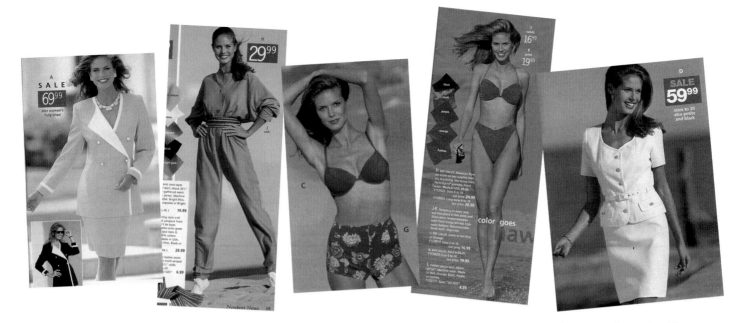

It was in my catalog days that I perfected the modeling "two step": two steps forward, two steps back, in a fake walk that was about as convincing as my smile.

Too bad Elite didn't share my enthusiasm. Originally they had promised me they'd take my career in a different direction, but it never happened. By now, the baby fat had drained from my face and my body was filling out. I was becoming a woman. I was the star of Newport News. If a piece of clothing wasn't selling on anyone else, they'd put it on me and it'd sell like hotcakes. (Once I was on the cover in a bathing suit, and when we all had a look at it, the team started crowing, "*Sports Illustrated*, eat your heart out!")

I know that not everyone reading this is an aspiring model. Probably not even most. But I think that this lesson could be valuable to *anyone,* in any profession or walk of life:

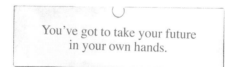

You've got to take your future in your own hands.

No one else is going to do it for you. You have to see clearly who you are, where you want to go, and what you can do to get there. Maybe it will never work, but if you don't try it yourself, you'll never know—and you'll never even stand a chance.

So I decided to follow my own advice. I told Elite I wasn't happy. (That usually scares them into thinking you're going to leave.) Even though I wasn't a big famous model, if I left, I'd take all my clients and all those hefty commissions. So they set up a meeting.

"Heidi, what's the problem?" they asked.

"What's the problem? I want to see better photographers," I said. "I want to do fashion shows. I've been with you for two years and nothing has happened."

"You're not a show girl," they said. And it was true, I wasn't. I was too curvy. I wasn't edgy enough.

So I said, "Look, everyone is telling me, 'You could be doing Victoria's Secret. With the body you have you could even be doing *Sports Illustrated.*'"

"Yeah, but they only use big girls." ("Big" is code for famous.)

"I'm tired of you guys always telling me that," I countered. "The only thing I'm asking you is to get me in to see the people at Victoria's Secret. Whatever happens after that is my problem. But I've waited long enough. I want *them* to be the ones to tell me I'm not good enough."

My agents got me a meeting. (It wasn't that difficult because, after all, agents use a quid pro quo: "If you want that girl, you have to see this one.") When I got to Victoria's Secret, I showed them my book. They looked at it and told me to change into some lingerie. I'd passed the first test!

My heart was thudding. I went into the bathroom and I put on their bra and panties, which fit me perfectly. They took some Polaroids and promised I'd hear from them very soon. When I hit the street, I went to a phone booth and called my agency. I guess Victoria's Secret meant *very* soon. "You're going on a trip with Victoria's Secret!" shouted my agent, who'd just gotten off the phone with them, "to Mustique with photographer Marc Hispard!" "You're kidding me?!" I was screaming on the street.

When I got to Mustique, I saw that Eva Herzigova, the renowned Guess? model, was on the job with a few other models I recognized. All of a sudden, here I was with the big girls. I spent the whole time studying what they did. I knew Marc Hispard was a great photographer, so when it was my turn, I just let him direct me. At first it was intimidating. The girls, the crew . . . everyone knew one another; they all

## PEARLS OF WISDOM

I've often found it useful, especially during stretches of professional or personal frustration, to think of my life as a long strand of pearls. Each precious little orb is connected to the next one, and to the next. Let's say each pearl represents a desire, or a goal to meet. The only way to keep your life moving forward is to seize life by the pearls.

How can this strand-of-pearls metaphor work for you? Envision something you really want to be or do, and make that the last pearl at the end of a strand. Now break down that goal into achievable steps on the path to that grander accomplishment—steps that you can take every single day.

All of these are pearls on the strand of success. And the great thing is, you can wear lots of different strands of pearls. Just as there are gray, pink, Akoya, and freshwater pearls, you may want to become an accomplished cook, a better friend, a mom, a skilled painter or singer, too. So, pile on those pearls!

Unlike the real thing, goals and dreams are free.

Nick Galifianakis

seemed to be a family. Everyone was looking at me, the outsider, skeptically—they see a lot of girls come and go before Victoria's Secret uses them on a regular basis.

I had to remind myself that it was a catalog shoot—and, after all, wasn't I the Catalog Queen? In this case, though, the stakes were much higher. Stephanie Seymour did this catalog. So did Elle MacPherson, Claudia Schiffer, and Frederique van der Wal.

We shot on the beach, and I felt at ease in my element. I knew how to work my hair in the wind. I knew enough to splash the water when I walked in it, to generate just the right fun-in-the-sun feeling. The session went well. We did only five shots—it would have been too much of a risk to put ten outfits on me, stick them in the catalog, and hope that they sold. But inside I was quaking because I really wanted this to work out. I wanted to be part of the Victoria's Secret family.

On a tip from a friend—and a hunch—shortly after I got back, I called up an acquaintance named Desiree Gruber, a publicist.

"Desiree, what is it that you do exactly?"

"I help people to get better known in their business," she said. "I work up little stories about them and share them with the press."

I asked her if she thought she could do something for me. "I just started modeling with Victoria's Secret," I said.

"Hmm . . ." she said. "What else?"

"There's nothing else really," I admitted. I had one tiny little straw that I could do something with.

"Okay," said Desiree. "We can try and make something happen."

One of my first Victoria's Secret print campaigns. I soon learned that Victoria *always* wears her heels to bed.

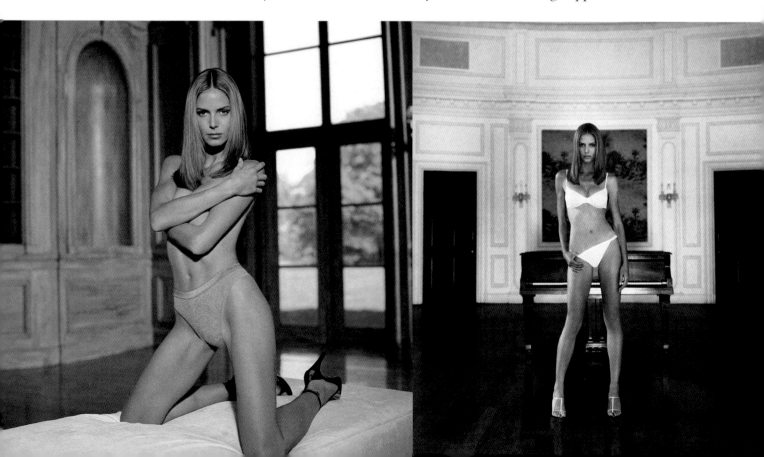

Being tapped to do the live Victoria's Secret fashion show was my next step. Of course, the company would be using their "big" girls—Stephanie, Claudia, Naomi Campbell, Helena Christensen, Tyra Banks, and Laetitia Casta. I'd done a couple of small, no-name shows—new designers that needed a model—in front of a small audience. But I hadn't done anything big, or anyone recognizable.

So when I showed up at the casting and they asked me if I'd done shows before, I . . . lied. I said I had. "Okay," they said, "show us a sexy walk. Turn at the end of the hallway and come back."

I knew they wanted to see that I had enough attitude to connect with a big audience. Plus since we'd be practically naked up there on the runway, we had to look proud and fearless: "Watch out or I'll walk right over you."

So I did. I strutted back and forth and smiled at them. "Great," they said. And I was booked.

Once I started working regularly for Victoria's Secret and got comfortable around Stephanie, Tyra, Daniela Pestova, and the rest, I hit them all up for business and career advice: How do you invest your money, or deal with international taxes? Can you recommend a lawyer? Who else do I need to help me? And, just as important, how do you always manage to get such great outfits for events? They had lots of good advice. Among the best? You have to be your own boss, and surround yourself

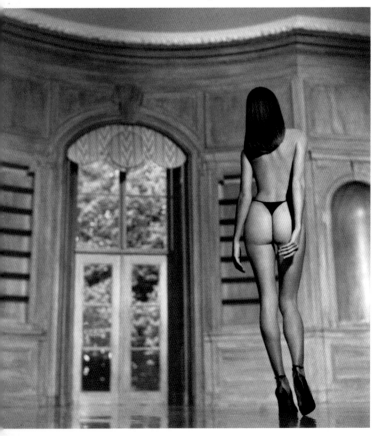

with a team of smart people.

I also learned just by observing. I noticed that Tyra always brought her own hair and makeup team because they were the only people she trusted to create this iconic person she'd become. She wanted to control who she was, rather than just being who a designer or employer wanted her to be. Plus I picked up some makeup tips. Her stylist would put false eyelashes on her or use some amazing hair product, and I would try the same thing on myself, with great results.

I quickly realized that if you don't make yourself into a personality, more than just a face, if you don't become someone that the public knows (or wants to know), then it's over for you pretty fast in this business. If the public is familiar with you, they want more of you. It may sound crass, but you have to make yourself into somebody in order to have a longer shelf life. Otherwise you're just the flavor of the month.

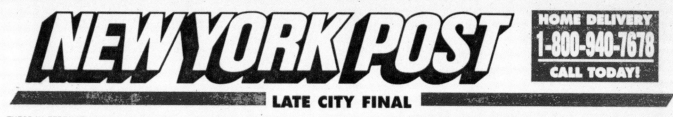

# NEW YORK POST

**HOME DELIVERY**
**1-800-940-7678**
**CALL TODAY!**

**LATE CITY FINAL**

TUESDAY, FEBRUARY 4, 1997 / Morning sun, 40-45 / Weather: Page 46 ★★R    http://www.nypostonline.com/    · · ·    50¢

# "THE BODY"

## Heidi Klum Takes Title

NEW YORK, NY— The night of my first Victoria's Secret show, I was terrified. It was to be broadcast live around the world from the Plaza Hotel, with a feed to the huge TV screen in Times Square. I knew I could walk a straight line down the runway, but I wanted to stand out and make the most of this opportunity. And yet . . . I was all nerves. Some of the most famous models in the world—Claudia Schiffer, Naomi Campbell, Tyra Banks—were roaming around backstage.

So my confidence wasn't exactly at its highest, especially when they let the paparazzi loose before the show started while we were getting our hair and makeup done. The photographers were taking pictures of every-

one but me, the new kid on the block. That's when my publicist Desiree did something that would endear her to me forever.

That morning, on "Page Six" (an influential gossip column in the *New York Post*), she had planted a photo of me alongside an item proclaiming that Heidi Klum, the new Victoria's Secret model, had taken over the title of "The Body" from Elle MacPherson. Now Desiree started shouting, "Oh, isn't that Heidi Klum over there? She was on Page Six today!" The music started thumping and we were all hustled into a line. All of a sudden, I was mobbed by paparazzi. The flashbulbs were popping and everyone was asking me what it felt like to be the new Body. Desiree, you're a genius!

My first outfit was this smoking hot black lace garter ensemble with a cape. I started down the

runway, with my head down and eyes averted, trying hard to vamp and look sultry. But my chin and little German knees were shaking. The runway seemed to go on forever. I felt a million eyes on me while cameras pivoted overhead. When it was time for me to turn, I did it flawlessly, but nearly wiped out on the way back with a double turn. All these tiny things a model does—the swings, the leg kicks, the hair flips—are what make her stand out. Naomi's the best at that. The more you do it, the more natural it becomes.

The next outfit was a cute slitted lace minidress, so I was able to call on my most natural asset: my smile. I beamed all the way down the runway. And that's what finally got everyone's attention— you don't see too many

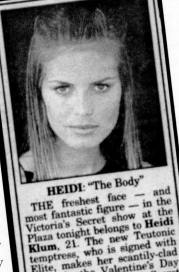

**HEIDI:** "The Body"

THE freshest face — and most fantastic figure — in the Victoria's Secret show at the Plaza tonight belongs to **Heidi Klum,** 21. The new Teutonic temptress, who is signed with Elite, makes her scantily-clad debut in the Valentine's Day edition of the Victoria's Secret catalog. The curvaceous Klum, who also stars in Givenchy's Amarige fragrance campaign, is being labeled "The Body" by industry insiders, usurping **Elle Macpherson**'s title.

girls who smile in this business! By my third outfit, I was having a great time, swinging my hair in my pivot and moving my butt as I walked. And then, as suddenly as it started, it was over. All I'd done was walk a quarter-mile in lingerie, but it was one of the hardest things I'd ever done in my life.

# yodelay!

One of the side benefits of being the new Victoria's Secret girl was that I got to do a lot of publicity, which gave a boost both to the brand and to my own career. My most important first public appearance was *Late Night with David Letterman.*

When it was time for the pre-interview, I knew I'd have to come up with some angle for my appearance. I had eight minutes. The producer was pressing me for ideas. I told them I could yodel, and they proclaimed it "genius!"

I came on that night in the most ridiculous outfit on the planet: a dress that consisted of little more than two pieces of black fabric, one in front and one in back (barely). From the side, it looked as if I had nothing on at all. Desiree was probably figuring, *Let's get her to make a real entrance and put her on the map.*

And the hair! It was as huge as Cindy Crawford's. David Letterman loved me. I was chatty but I stayed focused. I followed his jokes and dished his cheekiness right back at him. When it was time to yodel, Paul played the song I'd planned and I belted it out.

The audience went for it. Even David asked if he could get yodeling lessons from me. "Call me sometime!" I volleyed back as the segment came to a close.

The next gold ring to grab was the job I'd been coveting for years: the *Sports Illustrated* swimsuit issue. I put pressure on my agency to set up a meeting, and now that I had the Victoria's Secret gig they were a wee bit more cooperative. *Sports Illustrated* had recently appointed a new editor named Elaine Farley to plan the annual Swimsuit Issue. Each shoot is done in a remote and exotic location—usually, of course, on the beach. I brought her my portfolio and the Letterman tape, and she

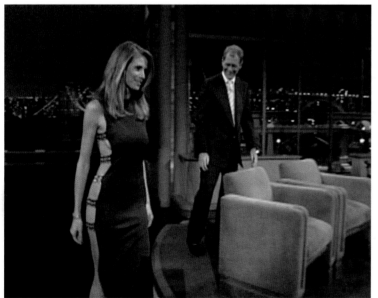

was brutally honest.

"I have to tell you, your book is not very good," Elaine said. "But I liked you on the tape, and I saw your pictures in Victoria's Secret, so I'm going to go ahead and take you with us to the Maldives." I was ecstatic! "But you've got to work on your book. It's horrible." She smiled.

I ran practically all the way home. I couldn't believe I was going to the Maldive Islands with Robert Erdmann, the great photographer, to do *Sports Illustrated.* This was the big time. So I went into training.

I started working out furiously and watching what I ate. I went to a tanning booth so I was sleekly bronzed, and I streaked my hair to look sun-kissed. I knew what came with the territory—I had to make myself into a hot beach chick with a rock hard body.

The flight to the Maldives was the longest I'd ever taken (and I hate to fly). But my nervousness ebbed a little when I got there and saw that Tyra was going to be on the shoot. She'd been on the cover of the Swimsuit Issue the year before; I'd worked with her on Victoria's Secret and loved her.

The first thing we did was fittings. I must have tried on fifty bathing suits. Then we did Polaroids and I could sense that Robert, the photographer, saw something in me. I think he related to the fact that I was a normal girl, sort of pretty but not gorgeous. He directed my hair and makeup, and made me look amazing. "I want you tousled and beachy, coming out of the water. I want you to be a goddess. I want people to drool all over you," he said.

It's a big deal to do *Sports Illustrated* for the first time. Even if you don't get the cover, millions of readers are going to know who you are. Understandably I was nervous. When we started shooting, I was trying too hard and kept overposing. Sometimes the best shots are the ones that look like you're relaxing on the beach and your boyfriend snapped a picture of you. So Elaine came over and told me, "Don't overdo it. Just relax."

We took some amazing photos that day. Then, as the sun started to set, Robert asked me to take off my clothes. I got really nervous. Practically every photographer I'd ever worked with had made the same request, and I'd usually say resolutely that nudity just wasn't my thing. But Robert explained to me that it would be a silhouette. The sun was going down behind me, so you could see the outline of my curves, but no flesh.

It's funny how you can become practiced at creating illusion. One of the best shots from those sessions is one where I'm lying partly in the water and my hair is slicked back. That halfway-in-halfway-out-of-the-ocean pose was impossible to hold, so I had two people on either side supporting my arms, and one person steadying my feet. My teeth were chattering and I was frozen stiff but thanks to the magic of photography, the three staffers were cropped out of the picture and I looked like I was just luxuriating in some balmy water.

Then Robert said, "Okay, let's do a cover try." Ninety-nine percent of the time, they do that just to make the model feel good. Nobody knows until the last minute who's going to get the coveted cover of the Swimsuit Issue. I certainly didn't think I stood a chance. But all of a sudden, looking through the lens, Robert got really excited. "This is the cover!" he shouted. And Elaine was going, "Oh, my God. I see it. This *is* the cover." Meanwhile, I was just thinking—remembering my dad's sobering advice—*Don't get your hopes up.*

I was back in the States shooting a commercial for Finesse shampoo when the call came from Elaine. "I have something to tell you but you can't tell anybody," she said. "You got the cover of the Swimsuit Issue." My mouth fell open. She explained that it wouldn't be announced for three weeks, though, so if word somehow leaked out, they'd have to switch covers at the last minute. When I got home that night, Ric issued an ominous warning: "Your life is going to completely change now. People are going to recognize you when you go out to get groceries."

## THE FIVE MOST IMPORTANT THINGS MY MAMA TOLD ME
BY TYRA BANKS, MODEL AND HOST OF *AMERICA'S NEXT TOP MODEL*

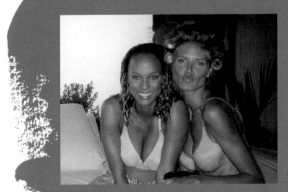

*Tyra and I bonded right away when we started working together. She's smart about her career, and, like me, she appreciates the value of good parental advice.*

**1.** Don't believe the hype.

**2.** Have a plan.

**3.** Look at the fashion industry as business, not pleasure.

**4.** Don't hide behind your representatives. Speak for yourself.

**5.** Wear control-top stockings when you wear white so they can't see the cellulite on your booty.

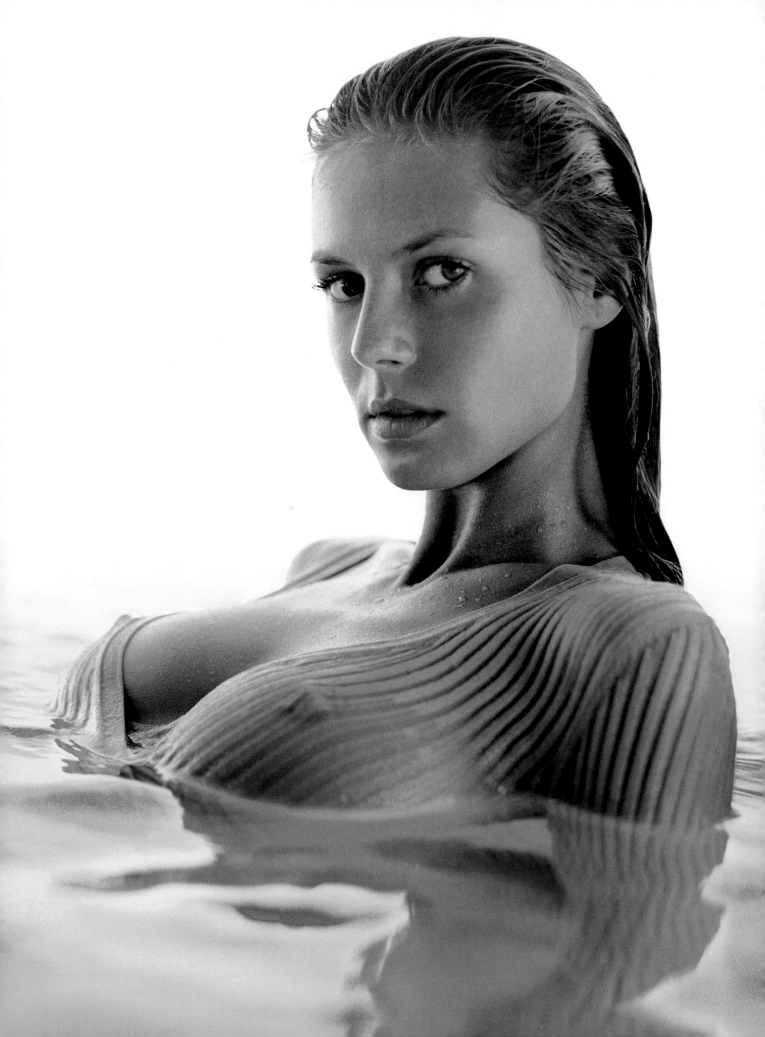

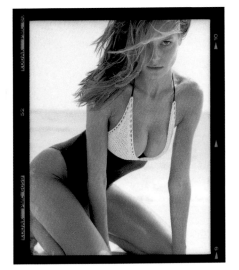
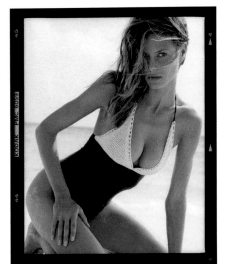
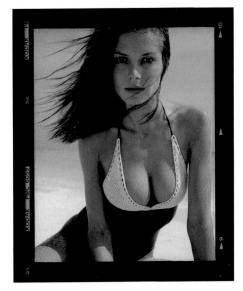
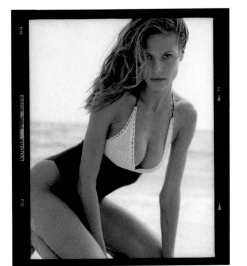
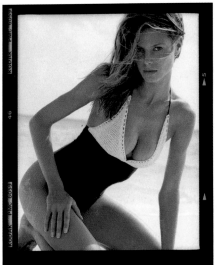
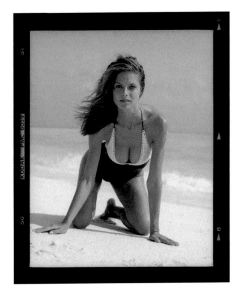
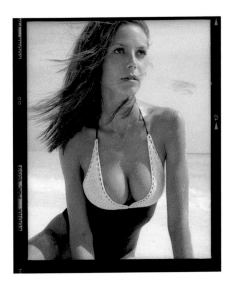
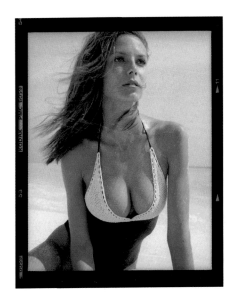
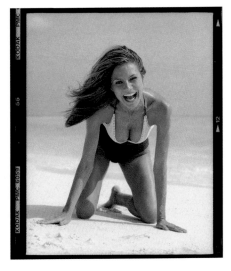

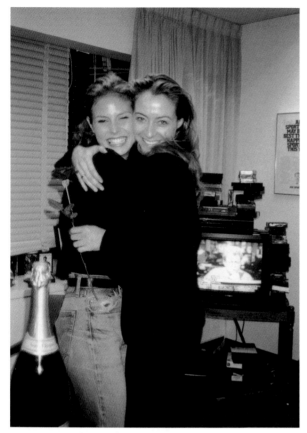

Then–*Sports Illustrated* editor Elaine Farley and me, right after she'd given me an advance copy of my cover. Little did I know how my entire life was about to get turned on its head.

Well, if the magazine cover didn't do that, the media blitz certainly did. I appeared on Jay Leno. I was a guest star on *The Larry Sanders Show*. I did *Good Morning America*, *Regis and Kathie Lee*, *Access Hollywood*, E!, Extra, CNN, MTV, German TV, Italian TV, everybody. I did a satellite media tour where you sit in a studio in New York and they hook you up with Bob in Tampa, Florida, and you ask cheerfully, "Hi, Bob in Tampa. How are you doing?"

I did twenty of those in a row.

Then there was the big party. I wore a beautiful gown, as if I were going to the Oscars. None of the girls typically dress up much for the *Sports Illustrated* party, but I was going for a glamorous look. I made Ric crimp my hair in old-Hollywood style with a side part like Betty Grable. My parents flew in for the party, where I did one press interview after another. It was exhausting. When we came home from the party, Ric and I lay in bed, watching a lightning storm roll in. I honestly thought there were people shooting photos inside the house. Let's just say it had been a long day.

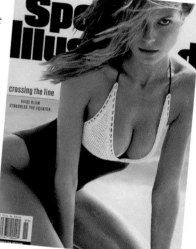

Then, as Ric had predicted, everything changed in the weeks and months after that. Eventually, too, I switched agencies and moved to IMG where I could have more opportunities beyond modeling: a bathing suit calendar, guest spots on TV shows, film roles, hosting awards shows, my own line of fragrance, clothing, jewelry, a video game. Whoever would have guessed what was in store when on a lark I clipped that coupon out of that fashion magazine back in Germany?

# just do it already

Life is so much more fun when you do what you want and when you can get your way, so long as you're not lying, cheating, or stealing to get it. (Okay, I'm not *always* an angel. Desire is motivating, but the other great motivator is revenge: Once in high school, my best friend Karin and I were walking home from school and some obnoxious kid was following us and taunting us with stupid names.

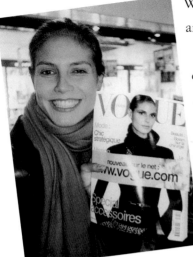

I did it—my first *Vogue* cover!

When we passed a dog run Karin and I spun around, grabbed him by the jacket, and shoved his face in dog poop.)

You have to be ballsy enough to go after what you want, creative enough to do it strategically, and humble enough to know that you can learn a lot by asking those who have more experience and wisdom. In my case, I've learned a lot not only from other models, but also from stylists, photographers, actors—even assistants. I've always tried to be nice to everyone I work with because the richest pearls of wisdom may come from unexpected sources.

If you don't ask, you don't get.

No one will reproach you for asking—whether it's asking someone out on a date or asking your boss for a raise you deserve. In fact, they'll probably find your confidence and bravery impressive. They may say "No" or "Maybe," but you will know in your heart what you can settle for. Just coffee. Or just a small raise. Or a let's-wait-and-see. From there, you can always prove that you're worth more, and keep asking until you get what you want.

## HOW TO BREAK INTO THE ENTERTAINMENT BUSINESS
BY HARVEY WEINSTEIN, COCHAIRMAN OF MIRAMAX FILMS

*The first time I got a sense of Harvey Weinstein's power was the year I watched the Oscars in my bathrobe and saw him walk up to the podium about a hundred times to accept an award for a movie he'd produced. I met him soon afterward. While some people in the business fear him, I think of him as a big bear, kindhearted and loyal. He's also worked very hard to get where he is. He gave me this advice for getting ahead in his industry:*

**1.** Seize any loose connection to the business that you have: Your cousin's girlfriend's manicurist's brother is an agent . . . who happens to be from the same small town as you? Don't be shy—track them down.

**2.** Offer to work for free—everyone loves a good deal. (Some ideas never go out of style.)

**3.** Go the traditional routes—they are traditional for a reason—and many are still effective. Work on a film set doing anything. . . . Start in an agency mailroom and work your way up. . . . Work as an assistant for someone you admire.

**4.** Read, study, watch movies . . . become more knowledgeable by doing your homework. Movies may seem like fun and games (they are), but they're also a business. As a doctor, you wouldn't go into surgery without knowing the difference between a patella and a pituitary. So you shouldn't go into a meeting with Martin Scorsese without knowing the difference between Fellini and the Farrellys.

**5.** Write and direct an unbelievable, groundbreaking first movie. Then call me (first). . . .

Most of all, good luck and always believe in yourself. My brother and I have overcome many adversities, and managed to come out on top because we believed in each other.

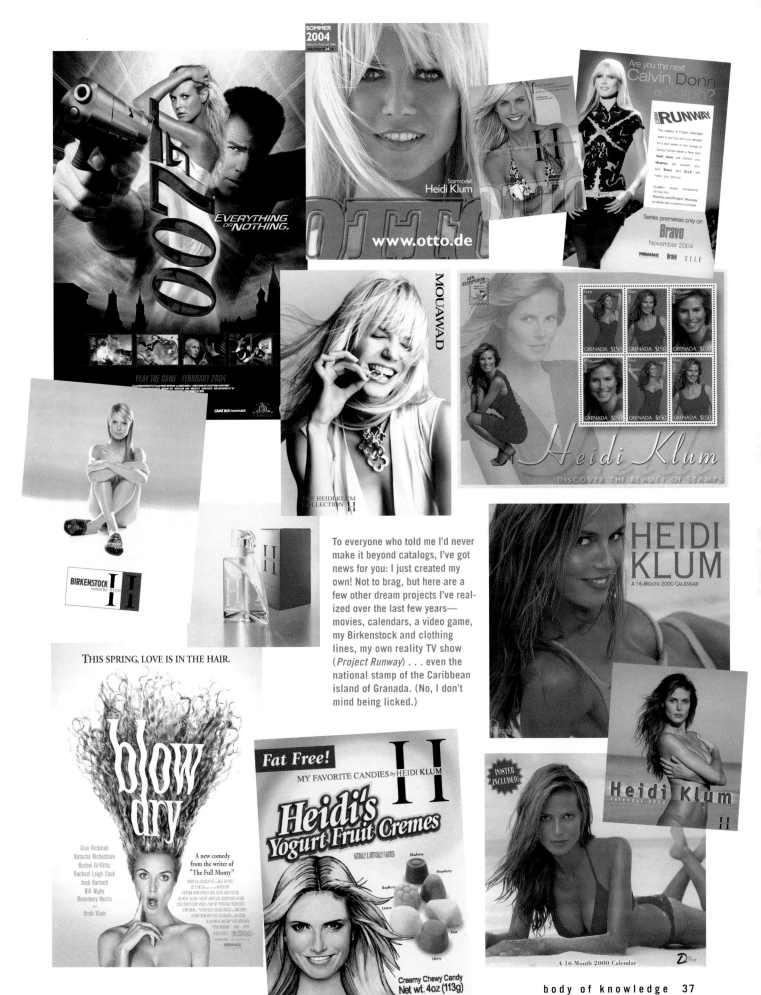

To everyone who told me I'd never make it beyond catalogs, I've got news for you: I just created my own! Not to brag, but here are a few other dream projects I've realized over the last few years—movies, calendars, a video game, my Birkenstock and clothing lines, my own reality TV show (*Project Runway*) . . . even the national stamp of the Caribbean island of Granada. (No, I don't mind being licked.)

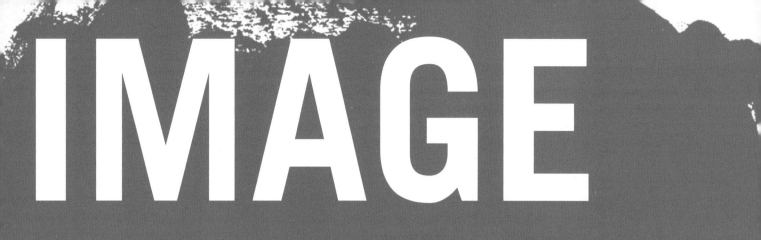

# IMAGE

RULE 2

*sell it!*

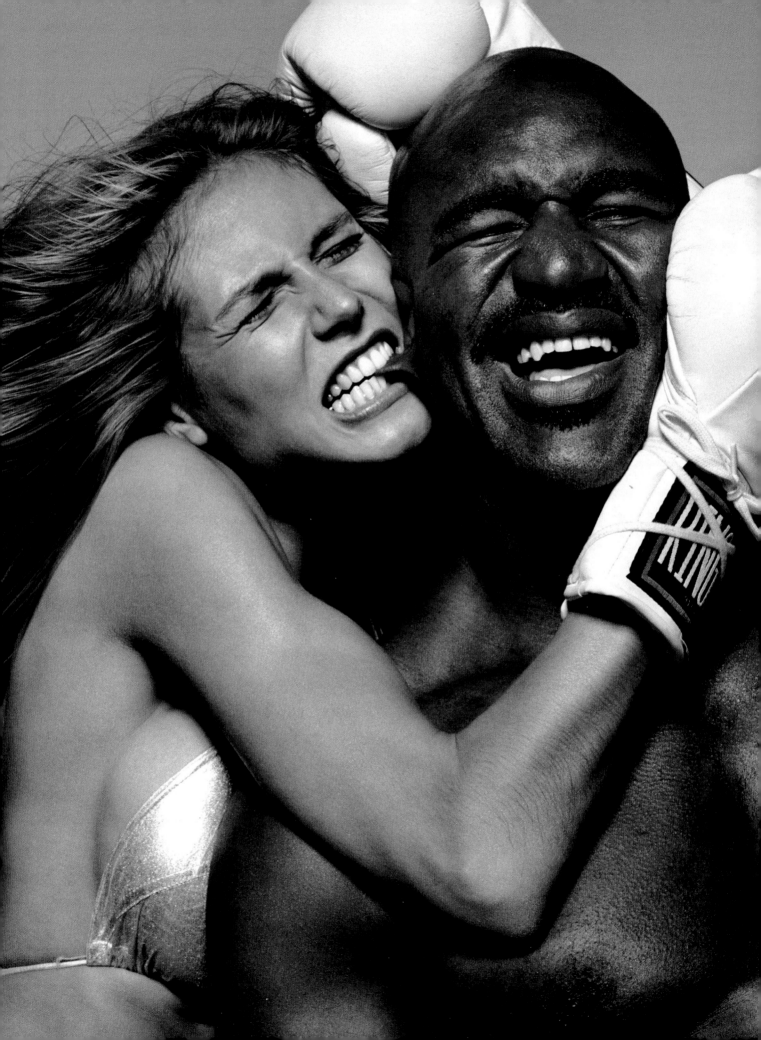

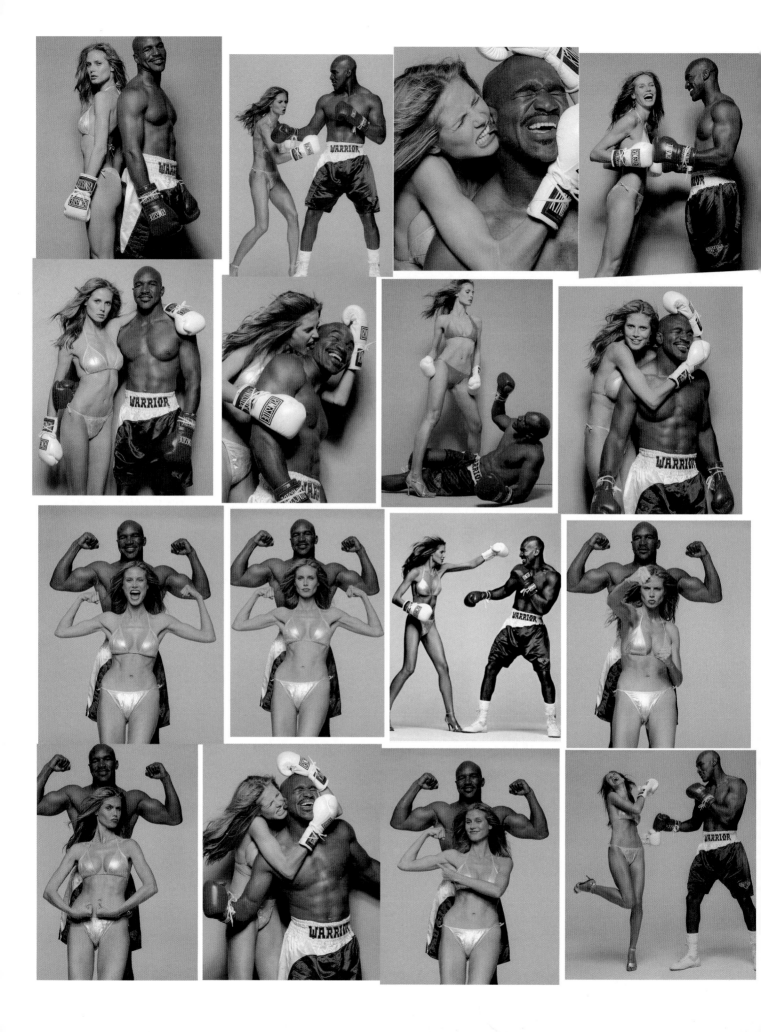

It was the morning of my photo shoot with then–world heavyweight boxing champion Evander Holyfield for the 2000 *Sports Illustrated* swimsuit issue, and the crew was walking on eggshells. A few months before, Mike Tyson had infamously ended their bout with a bite to the ear ("Iron" Mike was disqualified from the fight and suspended from boxing), and now everyone was nervous about how they were going to get Holyfield, this fierce fighter, to mug for the camera with a model.

Before Evander arrived with his entourage, everyone was prepping me: *He has to listen to his music! He doesn't have a lot of time! Don't ask for his autograph!* (Hmph, did anyone bother to prep *him* about *me*?)

But what did *I* want? I wanted an awesome picture, one that would be reprinted around the world, which sure wasn't going to happen if—as seemed to be the plan—The Boxer and The Model end up just posing next to each other wearing boxing gloves.

Actually, what I *really* wanted? Bottom line?

> I wanted to bite Evander Holyfield's ear.

I figured the way to do it was *not* by purring, *"Hey baby, let's make some great pictures together."* I think playing against type usually works well—or, at least, it's smart *not* to do the cliché thing. (Boxer = Tough Guy. Model = Sex Kitten. Yawn.) My best shot at getting what I wanted was by making Evander have *fun.*

So while he's dancing real slow to his Barry White CD, I started jumping around like a little Jack Russell terrier nipping at the heels of a horse. He's looking at me out of the corner of his eye. Clearly he's thinking I'm a nut. He started cracking up, dancing a little faster and shadowboxing me. I may have looked a little foolish but I knew the truth: *I'm* the one directing this show, *I'm* manipulating the situation. After dancing around for a while, I said, "Hey, Evander, how about you bite my ear, and then I bite yours?" The crew couldn't believe it—they were all off-set, peeing in their pants!

To everyone's surprise but mine, Holyfield said okay.

"But you can't laugh!" I insisted. "You have to look dead serious."

And so he did. And I did—*bite*—that tender right lobe. I grimaced for the camera. The photographer, Marc Abrams, got his shot, so he's happy. And I got exactly what *I* wanted.

For a man who's used to getting punched, Evander could never have anticipated what was about to hit him: I danced circles around him, I yodeled, I flashed my tonsils, I rolled around on the floor. All for a little nibble on what was left of his right ear.

(To his credit, the very agreeable Evander later said, "It caught me by surprise when Heidi bit my ear, but I didn't mind when I remembered that the last time someone did that, I got $35 million.")

In the previous chapter, you thought about your wants and desires. You promised to keep them in your sights on a daily basis. Now how do you make them into realities?

Hard work, yes. Dedication, yes. But just as important, you have to be persuasive. You have to persuade people that you have the talent, or the clout, or the creativity, or the sex appeal, or the sense of humor, to be the person you want them to see, or to do the things you're asking them to do. And you gain that power through selling an image.

That's the point of my ear-biting story.

## make-believe, and you can make people believe

Before the camera begins snapping, we models aren't exactly "on." Depending on the hour and location, we're either clinging to a cup of coffee or working our cell phones/BlackBerries/PDAs. But as soon as the music starts thumping and the shutter starts clicking, we know—if we're good at what we do—how to sell it.

What does "selling it" mean? I think it means *playing* at the person I want people to believe I am. Does that sound dishonest? I don't think it is. In fact, it's actually one of the hallmarks of successful people. Celebrities project images all the time—acting one way offstage, another way in the spotlight. Off the air, Howard Stern is a sweetheart; on air, he's the outrageous jerk we've come to know and love. That works to make him a success. Mike Myers is a zany man of many faces and voices, but in private . . . talk about taking it down a notch! Onstage, Prince (or the Artist Formerly Known As . . . or Once Again Known As . . .) is a charismatic, uninhibited talent; offstage, he's something far (*far*) more reserved. (Once, when we were both guests on *The Tonight Show,* one of his people came to my dressing room and told me that Prince would love to meet me. I went up to his room and we chatted for a bit. He seemed painfully shy. Then, as I was about to leave, I asked him if it was okay to take a picture with him. He asked me why I wanted to, as if it was the most outrageous request in the world. I told him that I collect photos of myself with celebrities, but he didn't think that was a good enough reason. "I don't believe in photographs," he said. "When I take a picture it's like something has been taken away from me." *Okaaay . . .*)

This ability to project an image is a trick of the trade. If a photographer poses me on a bed and tells me to look sexy, I turn into an enchantress, beckoning to some-

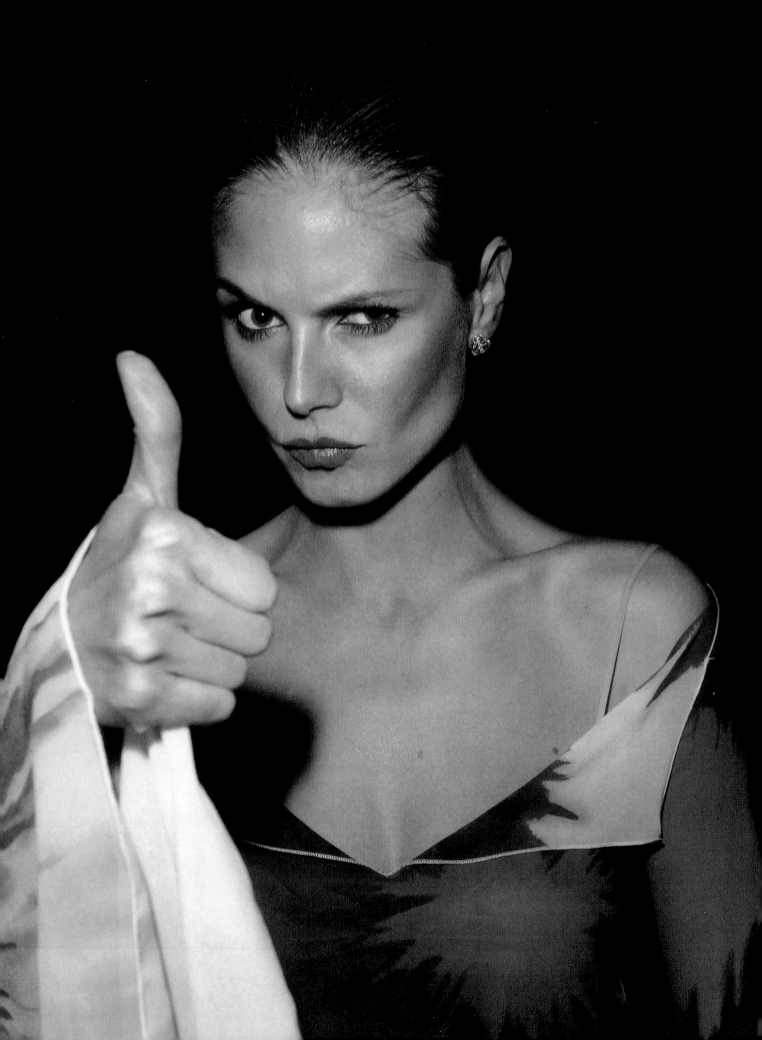

one just off camera. Or, more accurately, I become an actress *playing* that siren. If I'm supposed to do classy, I imagine Audrey Hepburn in *Roman Holiday,* or anyone painfully royal. If I'm supposed to be strong, I think of a James Bond girl: not necessarily the one who ends up with 007, but the one who jumps out of helicopters, flips off cliffs, and generally kicks ass. That's my Ultimate Woman.

Creating a persona that seduces—and I don't mean "seduce" in the sexual way, though of course that's part of it—can work whether I'm courting a client, meeting new people, or firing from all cylinders for a public appearance.

> "Selling it" requires a dose of make-believe.

But rather than think of it as a big performance that makes you all nervous and fearful that you'll fail and be exposed, think of it as playacting—something that can be fun to pull off, not to mention rewarding. The more fun you have, the more you'll let go. The more you let go, the more convincing you'll be—because you'll no longer be acting. On photo shoots, I've gotten so good at flirting with my eyes, for example, that I can do it even when I'm really thinking about what I want for dinner.

Selling it—and selling it well—takes practice. Before my first Victoria's Secret fashion show (which was to be broadcast around the world from New York's Plaza Hotel—yikes!), I'd never once done runway. And yet, in the weeks leading up to the

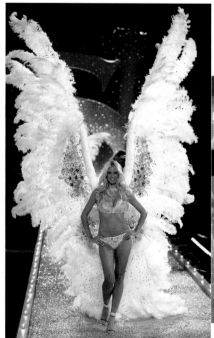

Some girls complain about the wings, but I love them—and I always make sure to get a good pair.

event, I knew I wasn't going out there behind Claudia and Naomi without knowing what I was doing. So Ric said, "Okay, we're going to train you." Good idea. I could focus on that. I could calm my fear (some of it, anyway) by actively *working* at something, and reduce

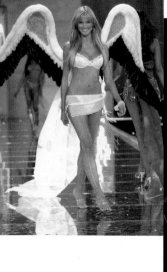

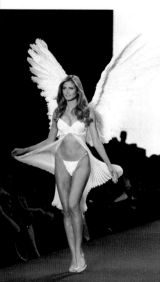

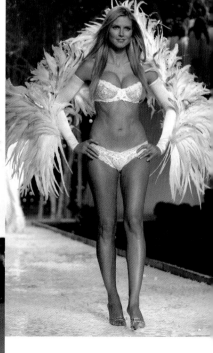

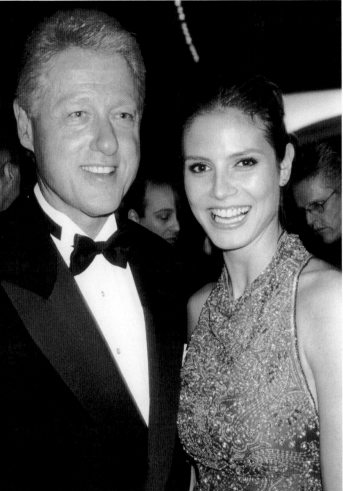

the number of things that were unfamiliar to me, for what was to be the world's biggest fashion show.

First, I went down to one of those outrageous boutiques in Greenwich Village where the drag queens get their outfits, and I bought a pair of super-high, glittery heels: good mood setter. Then I watched video after video of fashion shows to study how the models walked, moving their torsos and their bottoms like kitty cats. Now, I'm not really a super-sexy girl. Not that I'm a tomboy who burps and drives a truck, but I don't instinctively behave—or walk—like a woman. But to walk the runway, you have to have a sexy spark. So I tried it. At the time I was living in a railroad apartment, so I shoved all the furniture to the side. Wearing only lingerie and my towering heels, I paraded back and forth, from one end to the other, while Ric critiqued, telling me I was moving my shoulders too much, or not picking up my feet.

When it was finally showtime, I was nervous as hell, but I did great by just *pretending* I knew what I was doing. And, surprisingly, I kind of did!

Celebrities and other public figures "act" all the time. When I met Bill Clinton at the annual Correspondents' Dinner in Washington a few years back, the first thing I noticed was that this guy had an *aura.* He looks you in the eye like there's no one else in the room, as if he's the Wizard of Oz and he's going to grant you your ultimate wish. You can't believe how hard he's listening (or seeming to!) to every word you're saying.

Donald Trump acts confident no matter what the circumstances. Once, The Donald invited me to go to the U.S. Open tennis championship with him. During a changeover, his image flashed up on the big screen, and the whole stadium booed. I was mortified. But he didn't even twitch a muscle. He didn't care. Trump has learned to walk through life with his head up, secure enough in his own opinion of himself not to bother with what others think of him. And he's been broke twice! That's power (partly) because that's attitude.

There's a story I once heard that makes this point well. Marilyn Monroe was walking down the street with a reporter who observed to his amazement that no one was recognizing her. "Oh," Marilyn replied, "that's because I'm not being *her.*" And right there on the street, she transformed herself: *She became Marilyn.* Her posture changed, and suddenly, as if mystically, people paid attention to her. The reporter watched as passersby whispered and pointed, recognizing the great celebrity in their midst.

(I recently had an anti-Marilyn moment. Tyra Banks and I were doing promos for the Victoria's Secret show on CBS, and I walked in and the security people looked me up and down and asked, "Hair or makeup?" I said, "Uh, model." They didn't recognize me because I looked nondescript when I walked in, but once they did my hair and makeup, I became the Heidi they all knew.)

# nice girls—and guys—*can* finish first

If acting "in character" is key to selling an image, then first—and second—impressions count hugely in the building of that image. Too often, though, people think they have to be obnoxious to seem successful, so they act like jerks. That may earn you attention and intimidation (a poor imitation of admiration), but it won't get you lasting respect and goodwill. These are a few tactics I rely on for making a good first impression. Use them and you'll have them at "hello."

• *Be on time.* Who wants to work with someone who's chronically late? Tardiness isn't the prerogative of the powerful—it's just plain rude.

• *Shake hands like you mean it.* A firm handshake says you're confident and competent.

## HOW TO KEEP A POSITIVE OUTLOOK AFTER A SETBACK
BY DEREK JETER, SHORTSTOP FOR THE NEW YORK YANKEES

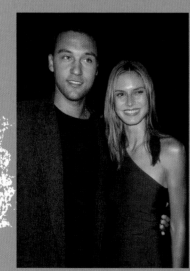

*I met the New York Yankees star shortstop when we did* Sports Illustrated *events together. He's a really nice guy, and famous for his resilience. Here's his advice for bouncing back:*

➤ Don't dwell on your mistakes. It's important to acknowledge your mistakes and learn from them, but you've got to let them go. And the next time you're in a similar situation, don't think about the time you failed. Think instead about all the times you have succeeded.

➤ Don't be afraid to fail. When you're constantly striving to be the best, you're going to have some failures along the way. Don't be afraid of this: It's part of what makes you stronger, and ultimately what helps you to achieve lasting success.

➤ Look to someone you respect for advice. Whether it's a teacher, a parent, a coach, or a friend, it's helpful to be able to talk about the setback with someone whose opinion you respect. They may be able to provide some insight into the situation, or just a shoulder to lean on.

- *Use eye contact.* It makes people feel you're focused on them and are listening closely to what they have to say.
- *Flirt a little.* It can flatter and generate a sense of intimacy—and not only with the opposite sex! But don't lay it on too thick or you'll just look like a tramp.
- *Smile or laugh.* An easy (and infectious) smile or laugh breaks the ice and makes you seem warm and receptive.

All of these gestures creating a positive first impression either put people at ease (good) or stimulate them (also good). And because you've helped them to feel good, they're happy to cede control of the moment to you. That's power.

Once you have that power, you don't want to lose it. That's where second impressions come in. To compare it to modeling for a sec,

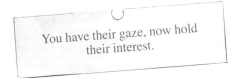

You have their gaze, now hold their interest.

- *Be a professional.* Treat people with respect and courtesy, no matter their rank or relationship to you. I always go out of my way to be friendly with assistants, stagehands, waiters, gofers, and other people who can be helpful to you because they'll remember it, and they'll be all the more eager to be cooperative.
- *Watch your mood.* If you're stressed or cranky or confrontational, your vibe will rub off on everyone around you.
- *Be organized.* Carry around a little book—I call mine my "bible"—that keeps track not only of your schedule, phone numbers, addresses, passwords, etc., but also of the thoughts and goals that come to you during the day.
- *Do your homework.* Whether you're meeting someone for a job interview or a blind date, find out something about that person, or his/her interests, or a subject that can be mutually stimulating. You won't be able to sound knowledgeable on every topic (when I sat next to Bill Clinton at an event in Germany, I can promise you we weren't discussing energy policy or peace in the Middle East—we actually talked about German food!), but if you ask good questions—and lots of them—you'll make a good impression. People just love to talk about themselves and their work.

I don't mean to suggest that by "playing" a role you're manipulating people. Or maybe you are—but who are you harming? And who's to say what's you and what isn't you? I'm a pretty self-confident woman, so was the nervous girl who didn't

## HOW TO FIND HUMOR IN ANY SITUATION

BY MICHAEL J. FOX, ACTOR

*Michael and I bonded during the taping of my six episodes for* Spin City. *He taught me how to act, he taught me how to kiss for the camera—but most of all he taught me how to make light of any given moment.*

**1.** Never take yourself too seriously, and feel free to find subtle ways to let the air out of any self-important gas bag you happen to run in to. Ask any little kid, there is nothing more fun than popping balloons.

**2.** Keep yourself entertained. You can do this by playing private mind games like "silent schmuck." I.e., If you are talking to a particularly exasperating person, silently say the word "schmuck" to yourself after every sentence. They'll have no idea, and it will make you feel better. I know my 14-year-old son does it with me all the time.

**3.** If you don't have faith in your own sense of humor, borrow somebody else's. What would the funniest person you know, a professional comedian, writer, or maybe your goofy uncle with the bad dentures and the whoopee cushion, think, say, or do in your present situation?

**4.** Always be on the lookout for irony: "What's wrong with this picture?" Is that Buddhist monk carrying a fly swatter? Why is there a "Greenpeace" bumper sticker on that SUV?

**5.** Seek out funny people and keep them close. In romantic situations a sense of humor is especially important. To but it bluntly: *Don't* f**k 'em if they can't take a joke.

**6.** Remember—one day you'll look back and it really will all seem funny. There's even a formula for this: Tragedy + Time = Comedy. Of course, there are exceptions, but basically: "That which does not kill you might just make you laugh your ass off."

know how to catwalk the real me? No. If you're at a party and find yourself stuck to the wall, too shy to approach people you might like to talk to (or even to give off signals that you can be approached)—is *that* the real you? Maybe not. So there's nothing wrong with playing at being the person you think will work for you, whom you most want to be.

## finding your best angle

What image do you *want* to project? If you're not sure, then notice how people react to you. What works, what doesn't? That is, what is it you're doing when you get a rise out of someone? What gets no response, or a negative one? It's different, of course, for each person. I see lots of models who do TV interviews or who guest-host shows, and they're good at it—but it's not the way I'd do it. When searching for your own "power persona," you can model your behavior on someone, but don't mimic them completely—it won't work. No one's exactly like you. See what feels most comfortable.

For example, in my business, lots of people act *faaaahbulously* sophisticated, *dahhling,* to get people to admire them and pay attention to them. I think this tactic is overrated (and overused). My M.O.? Usually I resort to humor. In fact, I act like a goofball a good deal of the time. I've learned that when I'm being funny and self-deprecating, people are more likely to listen than if I were to act like an I'm-too-important-to-talk-to-you celebrity. It's not always easy to be funny on your feet, but I try. When I'm a guest on *The Tonight Show* or *Late Night with David Letterman,* I always try to find a way to get the crowd on my side from the start. That way, *I'm* in control of the segment. Once on *The Tonight Show,* I waxed Jay's legs onstage, to make a point about how women torture themselves over their looks. I also confess to having teased Conan O'Brien's hair with hairspray into a shellacked cone.

To project an image, or to give people a certain impression of you, it helps to be creative and quick-thinking. Once, Tyra and I were presenting an award to rocker Steven Tyler at the VH1/*Vogue* Fashion Awards. As we stood backstage and read the script we were given, we thought, How boring! We didn't want to be just pretty faces reading the TelePrompTer. So we chucked the script and plotted something fun instead. When we got out onstage and began our tribute to the stylish and sexy-lipped auteur of "Walk This Way" and "Crazy," Tyra suddenly stopped, looked right at my boobs, and said, "Damn, mama, you look hot!" I took a step back, checking her out, and returned the compliment: "Damn, you look hot, too!" And with that, we threw ourselves at each other in a chest bump as forceful (and with as loud a grunt) as any professional wrestlers. (Tyra nearly popped me offstage!) The audience howled, and we made a much bigger impact (literally) than we would have as just talking heads.

Another time, I was on *The Tonight Show with Jay Leno* again to talk about the Victoria's Secret $11 million jewel-encrusted "fantasy" bra that I was wearing under my jacket. It was my tenth appearance on the show, and I'd once promised that to celebrate that milestone I'd yodel on camera. So Jay wheeled out a big cake and held me to my word. The band struck up a tune, I yodeled, and then for a finishing touch,

Tyra's my favorite partner in crime. When a producer backstage at the VH1 Fashion Awards told us to "Go out there and have fun, girls!" we did. . . . But we did it our way!

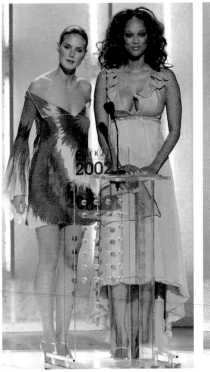
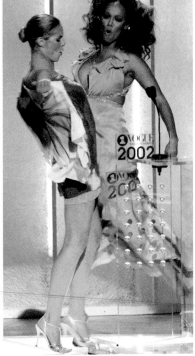

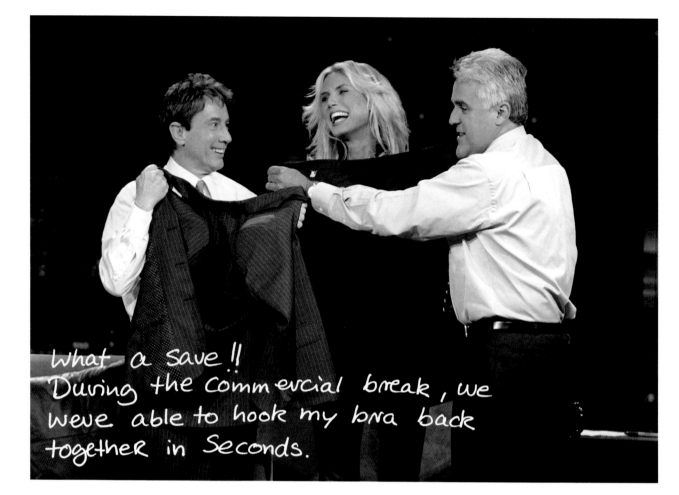

What a save!!
During the commercial break, we were able to hook my bra back together in seconds.

I decided to do a little "yelzin"—this scream we do in the mountains of Germany. I inhaled deeply—maybe a little too deeply—and boom! The bra broke. A few of the 3,000 diamonds spilled onto the floor (and my boobs came tumbling out of their harness). For a moment I panicked—how was I going to talk about the bra if I'd break the FCC regulations for nudity on television by showing it? I decided to go with the flow, so for two minutes (a *long* two minutes), Jay and Martin Short, who was also a guest, held up their suit jackets while I tried to disentangle the bra and bantered with them playfully about keeping their hands to themselves. I didn't get to say everything I was supposed to about the bra, but it got extra publicity because we managed to turn the episode into something people everywhere were talking about.

Doing something funny—trying to beat the script doctors at their own game—can be a blast, and has consistently worked for me.

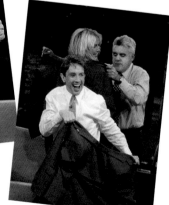

Humor can also be an antidote for embarrassment or stage fright. To get your mind off the fact that you're being watched or listened to by lots of people, you might start by imagining how nervous the next speaker is going to be, and find some entertainment in that. If I don't take big situations or famous people too seriously (or anyone who may intimidate: a boss, or someone you've been longing to ask out who you're finally talking to), I don't take *myself* so seriously, and I can relax.

Not long ago, I was in Germany to help christen the *Aida Aura*, the newest boat in the very popular Aida Cruise fleet. It was a great honor—Lady Di had once launched one of their ships. So of course I was pretty nervous. Plus, I was supposed to smash a big bottle of champagne against the hull of the boat, but not before reciting a five-minute speech I'd been given to memorize. Well, I'd learned it, all right (and learned it). I even had the paper on me, just in case anything went wrong.

The moment was approaching. I heard my name announced. I rose and walked to the podium. I was about to deliver my lines . . . when I blanked.

It felt like I just stood there mute, for five minutes (though I'm sure it was no more than a few seconds). Then, maybe without even meaning to, I made a joke— really, more a confession—of my fear to help me get out of my jam. "I'm so nervous, I completely forgot what I was supposed to say," I said truthfully. Everyone laughed—which gave me a chance to look down at the paper. And it all came back. (Making jokes, especially making jokes about yourself, can get people to be on your side, to root for you, to see your success as a good thing.)

## HOW TO USE STAGE FRIGHT TO YOUR ADVANTAGE
BY KYLE MACLACHLAN, ACTOR

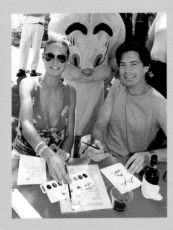

*I know Kyle well because he's married to my publicist, Desiree. He's perhaps best known for his starring role on the TV show* Twin Peaks, *but since then he's done lots of theater, from Broadway to the West End. The idea of live acting totally terrifies me! So I asked him where he gets the guts to do it.*

**1.** Nerves are good . . . up to a point. They can focus you but also undermine you. Even Tiger Woods is nervous on the first tee. It's his focus and prep that keep him in the fairway.

**2.** One great way to overcome nervousness is to practice your material in front of a mirror or video camera. You may cringe, but force yourself to watch till the end before destroying the tape!

**3.** Go over your speech again and again . . . and don't worry about looking like one of those crazy people who talk to themselves on the street. I once had a twelve-minute monologue that I practiced every night while walking my dog. I got some pretty strange looks—but it wasn't overly bizarre for New York.

**4.** When you're on stage, try not to focus on how you think you look or sound. Concentrate on what you're there to do. And slow down—speak more deliberately than you think you should.

**5.** The more you speak or perform in front of a live audience, the easier it becomes.

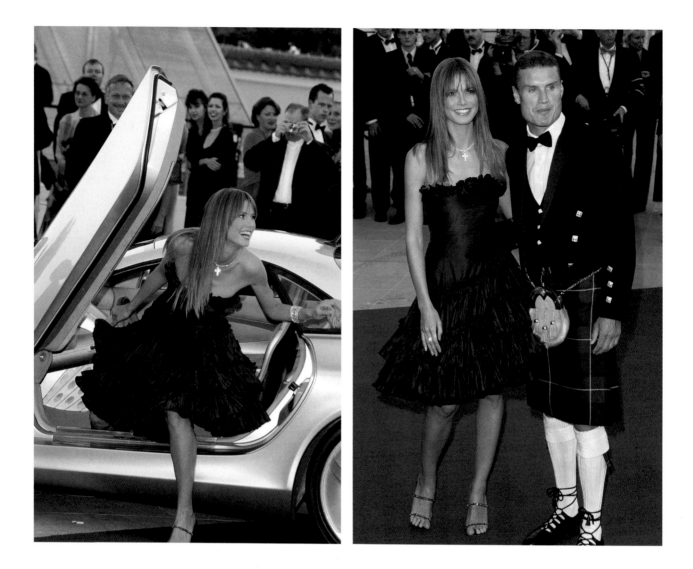

After insisting that I be the
one to drive Mercedes'
priceless new baby for a
memorable red-carpet
moment, all I could think
of was my mother's voice
saying, "Keep those legs
together!"

I delivered my lines, smashed the champagne bottle against the hull, and everyone had a great time, me included.

Then there was the time I was emcee at a sports awards show a couple of years ago in Monaco, and I was supposed to be driven up to the red carpet by David Coulthard, the professional race-car driver from England, in a $300,000 Mercedes prototype. But I didn't want to be the car babe—how unoriginal! Instead, I suggested that David ride shotgun, and I would drive the car myself. Well, the sponsors were wringing their hands, worried that I might crash their precious Mercedes. They even made me take a driving lesson beforehand. But in the end, the crowd loved it, and the photographs of The Model chauffeuring The Formula One Driver helped boost publicity for the event around the world.

You see, humor is only one way of projecting an image. There are as many different images as there are people. You just have to figure out which one feels most natural to you, and which gets the most favorable response.

# FROM PUNCHING BAG TO KNOCKOUT PUNCH: GETTING WHAT YOU WANT FROM ANYONE

BY JAY LENO, HOST OF *THE TONIGHT SHOW*

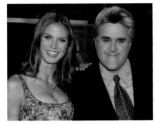

*I love Jay. I've appeared on* The Tonight Show *ten times and always have a blast doing it. What amazes me about him is his talent for getting even the dullest guest to sound funny and interesting, how he always knows what the audience wants, and, of course, that he has a snappy comeback for everything. Here's his advice for reading and persuading the people around you.*

➤ Always appear to be paying attention, even when you're not. Pretend what the person has to say is really interesting. (Hey, remember I do this for a living!) It's also almost always easier to agree, and if you can't agree, then at least pretend to agree.

➤ I guess this one applies more to women: Men don't really listen. Men just like to wait until you're finished speaking so they can speak. A real trick is, after you've said something to a man, ask him to repeat it—then you'll know whether he's really paying attention. Related fact: The more successful the man, the less he listens.

➤ In a relationship, there's nothing truly worth arguing about. If you're going out with someone who's sensible and normal, give in to things they really want; and if you really want something, they'll give in to you.

➤ However bad someone is on their best day, that's as good as they're ever going to be. I mean, if someone drinks and gambles before marriage, don't be surprised if they do it after.

➤ My attitude in life is: Look like a man, think like a woman. If you have a man walk down an alley and ask him what he saw, he'll say he saw a light at the end of the alley; a woman will say she saw two doors, one to the left and one to the right, a garbage pail, etc. Women have peripheral vision, while men just look straight ahead. Women are more attuned to body language, sizing up situations and seeing the whole picture.

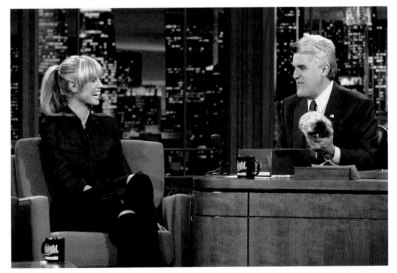

➤ If you're heckled while speaking, just turn the tables on them. Say someone yells out "You suck!"—just turn to the person and politely ask, "I'm sorry, what did you say?" If they do respond, it'll be with at least 50 percent less bravado and gusto. Inevitably, they'll trip and fall. Don't ignore the heckler . . . but if they've been extremely rude, be extremely polite back and they'll be intimidated. With the spotlight on them, whatever they initially said will sound specious and silly.

➤ When putting together a project, try to have as many diverse points of view as possible. Like on our show, we have equal numbers of men and women in supervisory/managerial positions. What looks like a cool guy to men may come off like a sexist pig to women; what looks like a sexy girl to the guys may seem trashy to the gals. Everyone working together keeps it honest. As a performer, I hate to play all-male or all-female audiences because then the point of view gets rude. A mixed crowd— that's the situation you want to be in. Most moderate change comes from the radical—you have people fighting for extremes and then you "settle" for moderation when you have different perspectives.

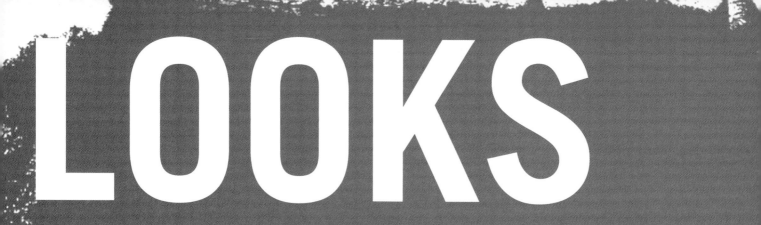

# LOOKS

**RULE 3**

*put your* best
face forward

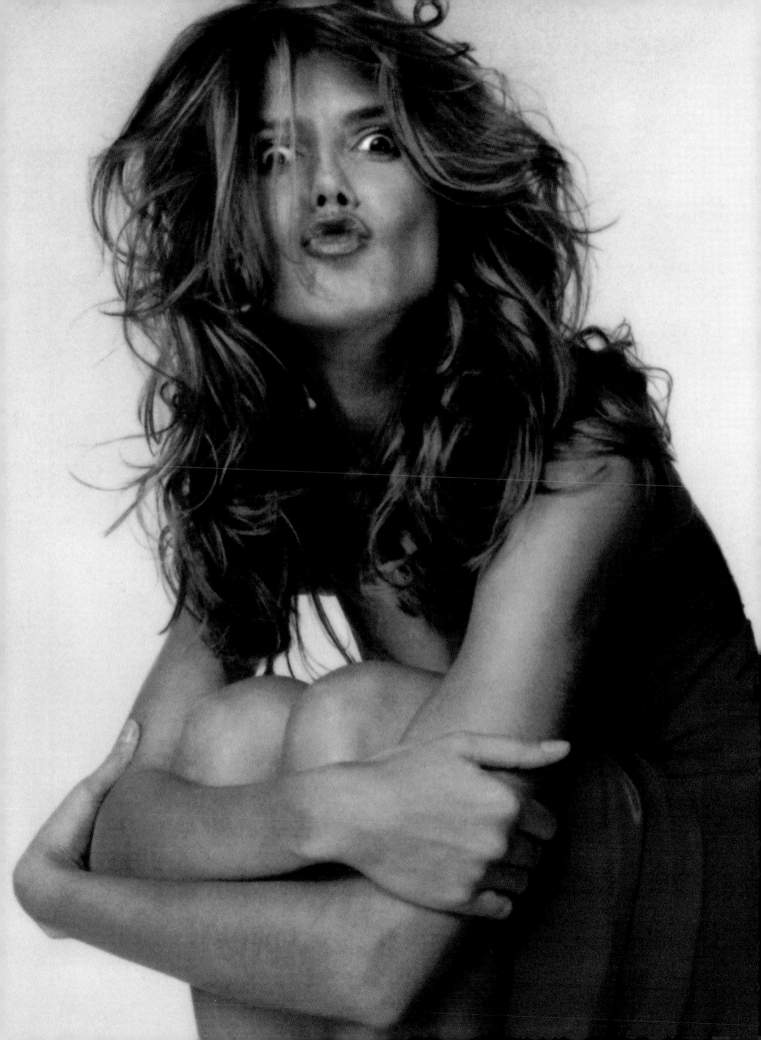

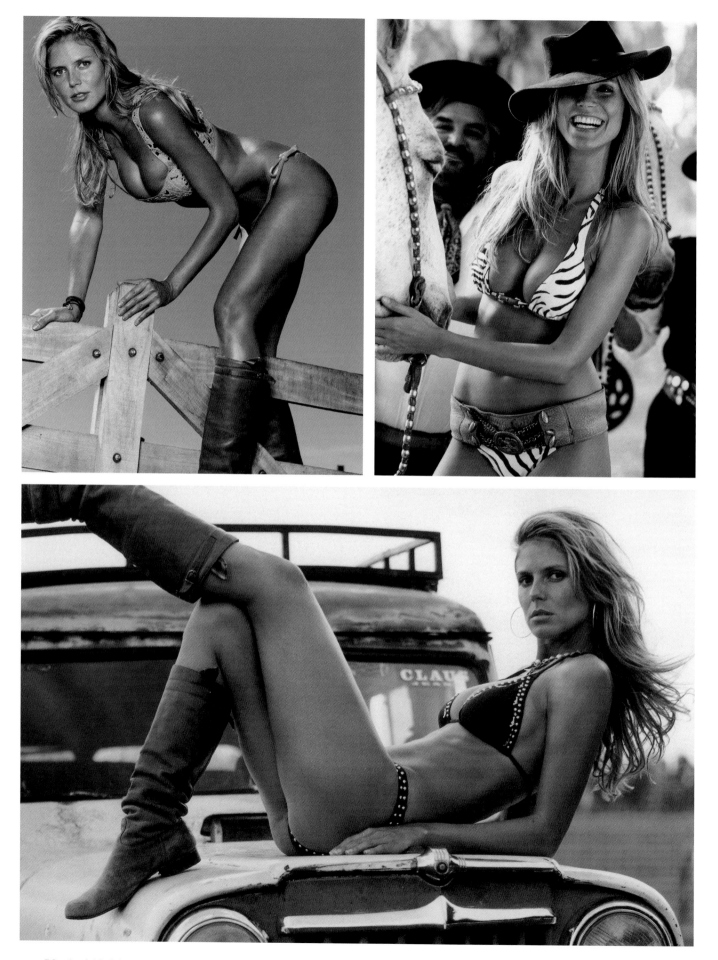

**P**icture the intimidating perfection of a model's face: the flawless skin, luminous eyes, beestung lips, bone structure so pronounced it could be drawn from blueprints, not a shiny strand of hair out of place.

Hardly.

The truth? It takes several hours and a fleet of experts to engineer a model's look into a beautiful portrait.

For starters, I've probably arrived on location from three time zones away, so that by the time I get to the shoot for the (not atypical) 5 A.M. call, I look like I've been on an all-night bender. Then, we get our hair done—a minimum of one hour of blowing, crimping, or gelling into submission. Next it's another hour or so of makeup to cover the blackheads and neutralize the dark circles to create even the most "natural," minimalist look. Some girls banish the red blood vessels in their

## LET YOUR BODY TALK: A FEW THINGS I'VE LEARNED ON THE BUSINESS END OF A CAMERA

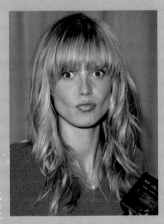

*Whether posing for a photo or flirting across a bar, you can create magnetism by tweaking your physical expressions. But don't overdo it—as photographer Robert Erdmann used to yell from behind his lens when I'd give him what I thought was my sexiest look: "Don't give me that stupid face! Just look at me normal."*

**1.** Smiling "inside" creates intrigue. Usually you show your teeth when you smile. But if you keep your lips closed, let the corners of your mouth turn up a bit (think of the *Mona Lisa*), and imagine your eyes glistening, you give off a mischievous, alluring vibe.

**2.** Turning your shoulder slightly, rather than squarely facing someone, can be flirtatious—not to mention physically flattering.

**3.** Arch your spine and keep your shoulders back and your head up to look confident (this can even make your boobs look bigger). Go too far, though, and you'll seem haughty and intimidating.

**4.** Sleepy "bedroom" eyes—relaxed lids and a softened stare—are sexy. Even more so if you're peeking out from behind deliberately touseled hair.

**5.** Keeping your mouth closed (you're breathing through your nose, obviously) helps you look relaxed and poised.

**6.** A slightly open mouth can be an inviting, sexy solicitation—but make like you're going to eat a blueberry, not a cherry.

**7.** Though laughing can create warmth, guffawing can make you look like an airhead—or a jerk.

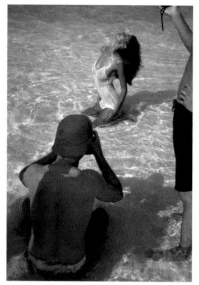

The making of a sexy photo: *It's just me and you, baby*—and about 30 other people making it seem that way. . . . After all that frolicking on the beach, I need a nap!

eyes with drops. Then we hurry onto the set, where the photographer has figured out the most flattering lighting using the beautiful morning sun, later blocking the glaring noonday rays with scrims so we can open our eyes (that's why you'll never see a squinting model). Between rolls of film or before setting up a new shot, a stylist will run out and adjust the flyaway hairs and touch up our lipstick or make us rosier with a dab of blush. (Even

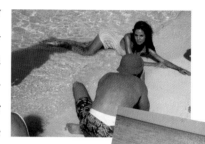

the poses are sometimes supernaturally sexy: For those oh-so-relaxed reclining-in-the-surf pictures, it's not uncommon for a bunch of assistants to crouch underneath you, propping up your back or pushing your hips out of the water so the image is as physically flattering as possible. The hardest part for all of us is trying not to laugh.)

We also owe much salvation to the art of photo retouching. (You should have seen the untouched first prints for a recent campaign I did for my jewelry line. I guess it's true that we are all our own worst critics, because when I was done marking the places that needed retouching, my face looked like it had some exotic black Sharpie pen version of chicken pox.)

The artifice extends to attitude, too: I've had to learn to turn up the wattage at a moment's notice and for long stretches of time. It could be freezing as I get spritzed down in my itsy-bitsy bikini on a winter's day, or it could be sweltering as I'm bundled into heavy wool coats and turtlenecks while the steam rises from a New York sidewalk. (Ah, the curse of fashion—that you shoot for the opposite season from the one you're in.) But it doesn't

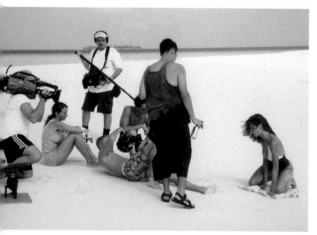

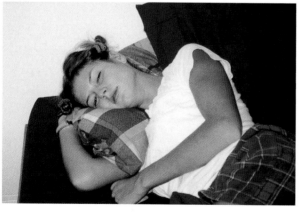

matter—I have to be smiling, sultry, sexy, sunny. And when I'm tired, irritated, or just plain nervous because there are so many people standing around scrutinizing my every pore, pimple, expression, and pose, turning it on isn't always the easiest thing in the world. It's hard to look all sexy, for instance, if your nose is running, your hair extensions are pulling at your scalp, and you're so hungry that all you can think about is whether you want pepperoni or mushrooms on your pizza at lunch.

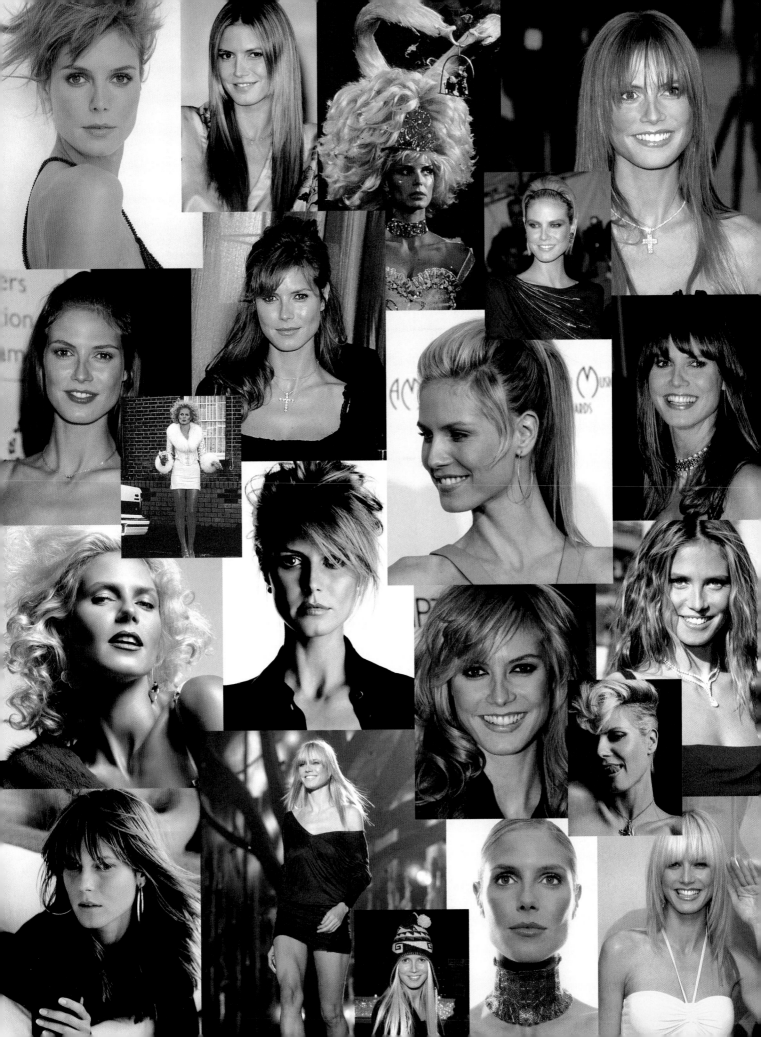

My point is that physical beauty, and the allure that someone projects through facial expression and demeanor, are all things that can be worked on, improved, embellished. Of course, there's no substitute for that real quality that draws people to you—charisma, sex appeal, warmth, exoticism, confidence, shyness—but sometimes it takes practice just to let go and allow these qualities to shine through, despite fatigue, stress, or a bad mood.

# the mirror has two faces (or three, or four)

We models make our livelihood from our looks—but to some extent you do, too. Sure, I could go on about the importance of inner gorgeousness, that beauty is in the eye of the beholder, blah, blah, blah. But inevitably, the way you look determines how people react to you (at least at first). Maybe you like that fact, maybe you hate it, but in our society, at least, that's how it is. You may glance in the mirror twice a day, twenty times, or not at all, but unless you walk around with a paper bag over your head, the rest of the world is checking you out constantly. Regardless of how you feel about your looks, the fact is that appearances matter.

> Your looks are your calling card to the world.

Whether you wear more makeup than Michael Jackson or have never been within twenty yards of a tube of mascara, most people do get stuck in a rut, looks-wise. It

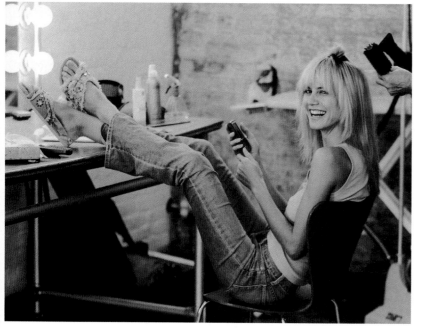

may be one never-changing look cultivated since college (if it's the one you had in high school, yikes!). The look seems to be working okay, so they do nothing to change it—whether they're indifferent, uncreative, or just plain chicken. They wear the same lipstick shade, maintain the exact same haircut and color, pluck those eyebrows to within a hair of their very existence. *Boring!*

Knowing my philosophy of life, you can probably guess my feelings about looks—that you should experiment, wing it, have as much fun as you can. No, not everyone will land in the pages of *People* magazine's "Most Beautiful

People in the World" issue (okay, yeah, I made the cut one year; Catherine Zeta-Jones, apparently the fairest one of all, got the cover), but you can play with your makeup and styling until you find a look that seems not only fresh but relevant to who you are right now and what kind of life you're leading, or want to be leading. Visit the beauty counter at your favorite department store—those makeup artists are falling all over themselves for subjects they can help! (Be careful, though: You need to be clever and resolute to get out of there with a fresh look but without breaking the bank.) Or ask a friend who's really skilled at her own makeup to give you tips. If you're carbon-copying the styles in magazines, however, do so at your own risk: There are only a handful of women on whom an opaque emerald green eyeshadow works—and they're all getting paid to wear it.

## MY SECRET BEAUTY WEAPONS

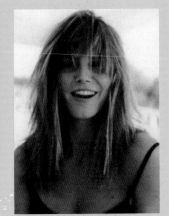

*Over the years I've gotten makeup pointers from so many other models and makeup artists—especially Charlie Green at Victoria's Secret. Not every look's a winner, but here are some tricks that have worked for me.*

**1. BROW BEATERS:** Most people pluck too much—you should really only tweeze the ones that are out of line. For arched brows, shape them with an eyebrow brush (I sometimes use a toothbrush). If you need it, use a bit of shadow or pencil to darken them. Then put a little eyebrow gel or hairspray on the brush, comb through, and seal the deal.

**2. PIXIE DUST:** Shimmer creams and powders (especially in gold) help you look dewy and fresh during the day, dazzling and seductive at night. Victoria's Secret makes a great one (this isn't a blatant plug; I seriously use it) that's contained in a brush—Charlie calls it her "magic wand"—which you just shake on wherever you want a little dazzle: on the shoulders, collarbone, and décolletage. Don't do too much shimmer on the face, though, or you'll look like a drag queen.

**3. LEG LIFTERS:** A coat of tinted moisturizer or oil can make your legs look tan if they're not, and more toned even if they are.

**4. LUSCIOUS LASHES:** I swear by my eyelash curler (make sure you get a good quality one). After clamping down to curl, you can darken the lashes at the roots with a well-sharpened eye pencil. Then brush on tons of mascara. For big Bambi eyes, use falsies (but you'll need the steady hand of a surgeon). Rather than using a whole fake eyelash, cut a strip into smaller pieces and glue a section at the outside of the eyes (you can also buy them precut into tiny bunches). Coat the whole lash with mascara, and hide the glue with some eyeliner.

**5. EYE BRIGHTENER:** Use beige eyeliner around the inner rim of the eyes to make them seem bigger.

**6. OIL CRISIS:** I always carry around little blotting papers so I can quickly stamp away any oil that seeps through during the day.

# play to your strength

Everyone's got a story about how, on the day of their high school prom, or hours before a blind date, or the morning of their wedding, they were aghast to discover a gigantic zit in the middle of their forehead.

But even an entire oily patch full of zits is nothing compared to the throbbing grotesquery I discovered once at 3 A.M. on a *Sports Illustrated* swimsuit shoot in Malaysia. When I woke up in the middle of the night to go to the bathroom and gazed groggily into the mirror, I saw to my horror that I had a big fat lip from what I could only figure was an insect bite. My mouth was so swollen you could see my teeth, so red it looked as if someone had slugged me in the face. Meet the next cover girl for *Ghoul Weekly.*

We had to postpone the shoot a day, by which time my bloodworm of a lip had gone from humongous to merely jumbo, and we were able (whew!) to downplay it with some genius makeup.

But the lesson wasn't lost on me: The secret to beauty is to highlight and hide. Highlight not only what you want them to see, but to the point that you've distracted them from what you *don't* want them to see.

> A bad hair day is another way of saying, "Today my skin looks amazing."

Everyone's got at least one feature that's distinctive, one that you can at least tolerate if not love. Pick a part and make it work for you.

How?

For instance, despite my Malaysian mishap, my best trait, I think, is my smile. It's quite noticeable from afar (I prefer the grin to the signature model smirk), so I don't really need gobs of lipstick. I just go with a light gloss, then play up my eyes with mascara, liner, and shadow. You can use the same trick to highlight a gorgeous mouth with color, bring out cheekbones, or draw attention to your beautifully colored eyes with a matching shadow.

Makeup isn't your only ally when trying to look your best. A cold sore is just an excuse to make your hair look fabulous. If allergies have made your eyes bloodshot, then throw on a colorful neck scarf—the eye of the beholder will go there first. And a bad hair day calls for a vibrant shade of lipstick or an elegant hat. All good visual artists—interior decorators, photographers, painters, pastry chefs—are skilled at making you see what they want you to see. That's what makeup artists do for us models, and what you can do for yourself.

# save me some skin

Models have some of the worst skin on the planet. Seriously. If you think about it, it makes sense: We're constantly being troweled with heavy makeup, pulled, plucked, glued, and forced to endure every abuse imaginable to our skin, including flying so often we get as parched as the Gobi Desert. True, we can be found most Saturday mornings treating ourselves to a facial, but hey—we deserve it.

The skin is the body's largest organ, so you should take care of it as you would any other vital body part. You know the drill: gentle cleanser, moisturizer, sunscreen even if it's a little cloudy. Sure, you can go the extra distance and max out on toners, firming creams, rejuvenating gels, alpha-beta-omega acids, etc. But I think that if you maintain the minimum, you'll be thanking yourself because when you're seventy, you'll be able to pull on your skin and it will actually snap back before the end of the month.

Another reason models have such skin issues is that (if we're lucky enough), we spend an extraordinary amount of time under the hot sun. I want a healthy, glowing tan, but I don't want damaged skin, year after accumulating year. So how do I

## LOOK BETTER IN LINGERIE
BY CHARLIE GREEN, VICTORIA'S SECRET COSMETICS GURU

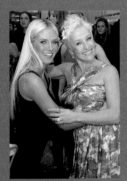

*I've been working with makeup artist extraordinaire Charlie Green for years. Anytime I have to do a special event, Charlie is one of the first people I call. She also knows more about creating a sexy look than anyone.*

➤ Slather yourself with body lotion from head to toe. It makes skin look and feel more gorgeous.

➤ Dust a very fine shimmer powder all over so you look dewy and radiant. Avoid silver or lilac tones, which don't look good on anyone; instead, go for the more universally skin-flattering shades of gold or peach.

➤ Add a touch of semi-matte bronzing powder to cleavage, to enhance your . . . feminine qualities.

➤ You can also use bronzer to define ab muscles or the area along the bikini line.

➤ Finish with perfume and lots of black mascara.

➤ Hit the dimmer switch.

keep a tan year-round? And why, even though I spend so much time in a bathing suit, don't I have tan marks to show for it?

I fake it.

Ah. It feels so good to confess.

It used to be that fake tanners left you looking like George Hamilton on a carrot-juice diet, but in the last few years, tans in a bottle have progressed to the point where they're nearly indistinguishable from the real thing. A couple of rules: Apply less where you would naturally get less color (backs of the knees, inside of the arms); avoid wearing white immediately after you treat your skin (unless you want the whole world to know that you're a bottle bronzer); wash your hands well after slathering on the stuff. (Ever seen anyone with tan palms? Me neither.)

If you can spring for it, try getting your self-tanner professionally applied. Many salons and day spas offer a version of the spray-on tan that's evenly distributed on the body and lasts a bit longer than the bottle tans.

# hairy situations

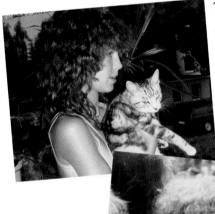

They say hair is a gal's crowning glory. And it's true—for a lot of people, hair is a major source of vanity, pride, frustration, obsession. . . . I've even heard of a study that says that, given the choice between great hair days or great sex for the rest of their lives, more women would choose the cooperative hair! And in my profession, there's no feature that models are better known for than their hair. Gisele's sandy bedhead mane. Rebecca's tousled blond corkscrew curls. Linda Evangelista used to change her haircut and color so often, the only look she was consistently associated with was the one she'd just shed (though it was probably the short, sharp-angled bob that people remember best).

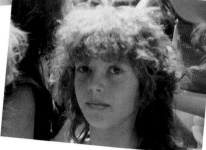

When I went blond after years of being at times an admittedly mousy brunette, people very straightfor-wardly said they liked me better the new way, that I looked happier and more relaxed— which made me wonder what else they weren't telling me! Because color change in modeling can generate buzz, I started getting considered for more diverse and exciting jobs. (Not that I think blondes have more fun —we just tend to be more noticeable.) Now, of course,

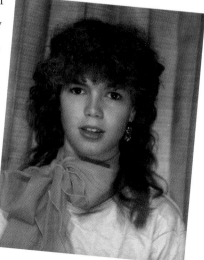

I've never been hesitant to try new styles—I mean, *I* thought I looked great in a poodle perm! I'm sure you can recall some of these looks, from the teased bangs to the rockabilly pouf. (I credit my mother with some of the more outrageous creations.) Who knows what I'll do next?

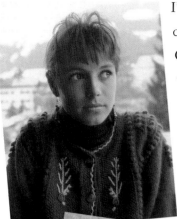

I'm addicted. Even though I was born to one hairstylist and married to another, I can't believe there was a time when I ever did so little to make my hair look great. Okay, so there was my "Nena" period in the 1980s (remember "99 Red Balloons"?) when I got a poodle perm, something my mother still won't let me live down.

For the purposes of attracting men, hair is like breasts: They think it's sexy and want to touch it. (Which is why models with long hair, in my experience, generally have more work opportunities than those with short hair.) Yet too often, smart women forget that maybe the most crucial tool of seduction is right there atop their brains. Whatever you do to it—color, fringe, radically chop it off—remember: *It's only hair.* It will grow out, grow back, grow into whatever you wish to do with it. So rather than be cautiously conservative, why not be a little more creative and daring?

Some lessons I've learned from the scissorhands in my life:
• *Wear your hair at a proportional length.* If you have a small head on a big body, you should have longer hair. (With my bigger frame, long hair makes my body look smaller.) Large heads only look more voluminous with big hair. You catch my drift.
• *Don't get the trendy cut of the moment if it's not "you."* If you're not into bangs and will end up just pinning them back all the time so you can see, don't bother getting them in the first place, because they take a long time to grow out. That hipster shag? Maybe best left to the painfully ironic and those on a prime-time TV series.
• *Play around.* Regardless of what type of cut you have, hair is versatile. Switch the part, wear cute accessories, pin it half up, half down, experiment with curlers and irons.

## time to change

How much time does it take to look better?

Very, very little. Sure, models are professionally motivated to spend more time on their looks, just as athletes are similarly motivated to spend more time on their bodies. But it's amazing how many quick tweaks we can do—or not—that can change how others perceive us.

Indeed, the most basic grooming and beauty regimen takes barely any time, and can yield great benefits in our looks-obsessed culture.

Try telling that to most men, though.

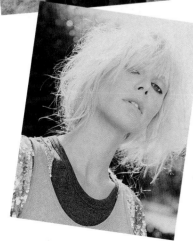

To: Men
From: A Secret Admirer
Re: EPIC MISTAKES YOU GUYS MAKE
Cc: Other Women
Bcc: Guys Who Don't Think This Applies to Them

You'd think it goes without saying, but what the hell: A guy should be nicely groomed. That doesn't mean you need to be pomaded and plucked and polished, metrosexual style. Nor does it mean there's one single look to aspire to, since no one style makes the majority of womankind happy (I love hairy chests, other women don't).

On the other hand, you need to show self-respect. And speaking of hands, can we start with those?

1. Nails from Hell: It's not just that dirty or chewed-up or overlong fingernails and toenails look disgusting. It's that they tell the world that you don't take care of yourself, generally--maybe because you don't know how, maybe because you simply don't care. Whatever the message, it isn't good.

2. Poor Teeth, Worse Breath: If teeth aren't clean and clean-smelling, then you might as well take every other good grooming habit you follow and toss them in the Dumpster because this is as nonstarter as it gets. You're not getting past this--or, rather, we're not. Smokers, of course, have lots of oral challenges. So either quit or be extra vigilant in the plaque and enamel departments (no, popping mints before a kiss doesn't count).

3. Scent: Elevators, sushi bars, airport security lines—they're all tight and crowded. Ease up on the aftershave and cologne, please. A natural smell is actually very nice and sexy--well, unless you've just run a marathon or are going for a world record in the wearing-the-same-shirt-for-days event. In such cases, take a shower . . . and then go easy on the aftershave and cologne.

4. Stray Hairs: That's right--not "hair" but "hairs." Unwanted dark hairs growing out of your nose? Bad, very bad. There's nothing else we see when we look at you; it's like spinach in the teeth, only way grosser. Ear hairs? Back hair the breadth of an area rug? Unibrow? Trim away!

5. Neglected Skin: If you can't take care of your skin by yourself, think about a facial. It's not a sissy thing; it'll clean out years of accumulated junk from your pores, and--no small bonus--it feels incredible. They'll even give you a terry cloth robe and supercomfy jelly slippers at the spa if you ask real nice, boys.

6. Vanity: Speaking of "sissy things," if a man spends more time in front of a mirror than I do, forget it. Don't misunderstand: I'm all for equality of the sexes. For men, it's important to be clean, better to be groomed, fine to be stylish. But here's what creeps me out: If a guy spends so much time looking at himself, what exactly is he looking for?

# look your best (in the photo album)

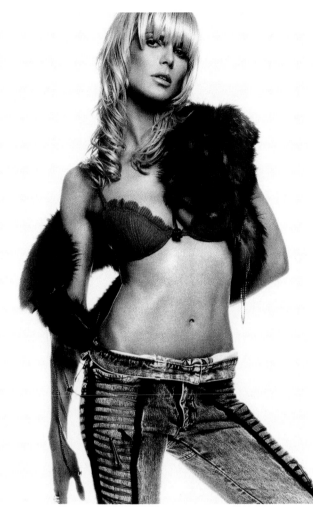

You have to be comfortable in your skin. Maybe that means a little face paint, maybe not. For the most part, however, models look their best in front of the camera by making their face appear as *natural* as possible. After a shoot, when I see the contact sheets, the best pictures are always the ones where I look the way I usually look (smiling, alert, relaxed), and the worst are those in which I'm making some weird face. Photographer Robert Erdmann, who takes some of the sexiest pictures that have ever appeared in the *Sports Illustrated* swimsuit issue, is always saying, "Don't give me that stupid face. Just look at me normal."

Your "normal" is something only you can determine. Maybe it's *not* smiling; maybe it's a sultry gaze. Certainly, billions upon billions of home photographs have been degraded by having everyone fake-smiling "Cheese!" for the uncreative photographer (mom, dad, annoying uncle). I find the best ways to try to look like you're *not* trying are:

- Pretend you're starting a conversation rather than getting "ready" to take a picture
- Look at a point past the camera and imagine the lens isn't there
- Relax your facial muscles. No cheek bunching!
- Try to think of something pleasant or funny and react to it

My point is that ultimately, an idealized version of "normal" is what you want to look like in every situation. Even if you get a professional makeover, you still want to look like *you* when it's done, with your most admirable qualities shining through: your sense of humor, your intelligence, your affability. Still, there may be another version of you—a more glamourous, elegant, bohemian, romantic, or vixenish you—waiting to find expression. I think it's time you had some fun discovering just who the new you (or yous) might be.

# STYLE

**RULE 4**

*make a* fashion statement

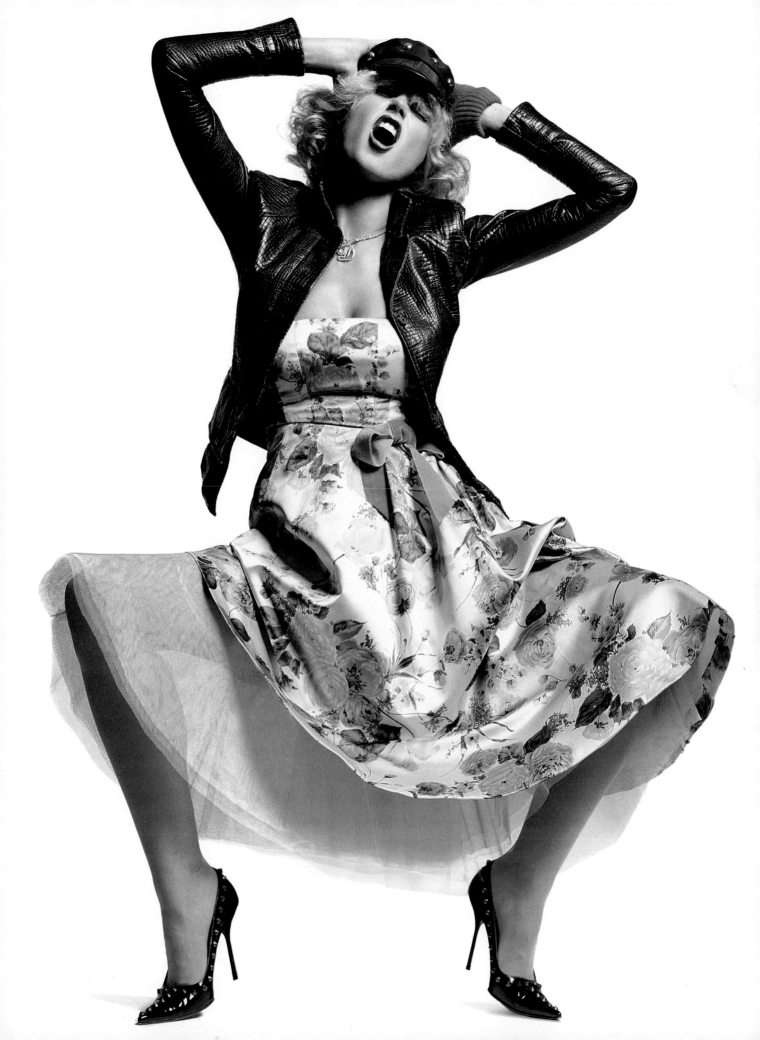

It may seem as if models have an innate sense of style: We wear all the up-to-the-minute couture and ready-to-wear designs months before they appear in magazines or stores, and they fit us so well we could have been born in them. When we're photographed at parties and premieres, we can pull off the most breathtaking designer creations with nonchalance, as if we're wearing nothing more complicated than jeans and a T-shirt: *Oh, this tulle thing? I found it in my laundry hamper. . . .*

While some models do have a natural eye for design or have cultivated a unique personal style, most of us need a certain amount of assistance to look the way we do. For one thing, it's likely we've been taped, pinned, padded, and sewed into whatever we're wearing on the runway, in a magazine, or on the red carpet. For another, it's not exactly a secret that most of the photos of us that land on party or gossip pages feature outfits we've borrowed from designers. We get to look like Cinderella for an evening, but when the clock strikes midnight (okay, more like 3 A.M.), we have to give it all back. Sometimes there's even a celebrity or stylist in another country who has reserved that very dress—the exact same one-of-a-

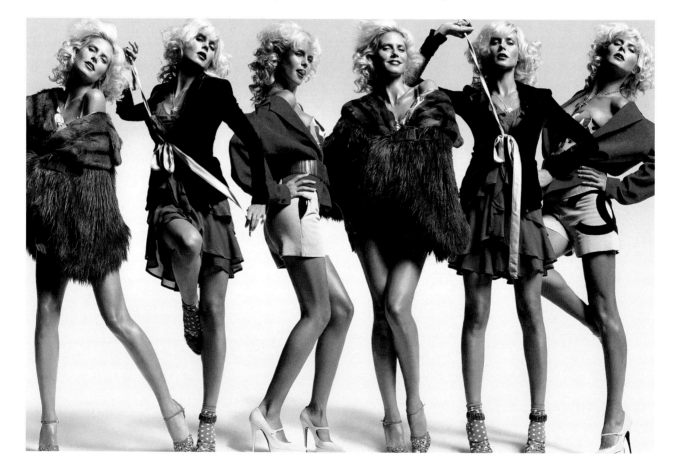

kind creation, lipstick stains and all—to be shipped to them for use the next day, and the dress embarks on a world tour, like some kind of rock star.

# once upon a style

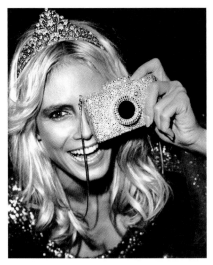

I've always loved playing dress-up, and it used to be that to call my style flashy wouldn't have been a stretch. After making it onto one too many "worst-dressed" lists in the States, where tastes are somewhat more conservative than in Europe, I realized I needed help.

So I hired a really great stylist named Rachel Zoe Rosenzweig, who lives in Los Angeles and works with many celebrity clients. When I first called her, I wanted to be more fashion-forward without becoming a fashion victim. What does that mean? Adapting the current trends to who I really am.

Having said that, I'm definitely not styled and in the latest looks all the time. There's a big difference between dressing "nice" for a normal dinner party and "fabulous" for a fashion-centric dinner party. (Besides, there can be hazards to looking too fashion-y. How many times have I squeezed into the perfect dress, tempting fate? Like the time I was in the limo on the way to the *Sports Illustrated* swimsuit issue party: I had primped and preened and gotten the *perfect* dress. I'm not going to name the designer because I still love him, but all the hooks and straps pretty much started coming apart. I don't mind the deconstructed look, but not *that* much. My publicist ended up having to safety-pin me together and do spot checks for boob slippage the whole night!)

But how do you determine *your* style? What can work for you on a daily basis, when you're more likely to face colleagues at work or friends at school than a throng of paparazzi and judgmental fashion police? Unless you've been living in a nudist colony your entire adult life, you have some sense of the looks you're comfortable in, the colors that flatter, the silhouettes that fit best.

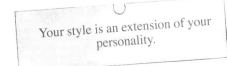

Your style is an extension of your personality.

That may translate to a fashion sense that is reserved, edgy, romantic, earthy, playful, or sporty. Or it may be three of those, at different times of the day or week. Clothing is such an easy way to define an image, to help you project whatever it is you want the world to understand about you. (Don't go overboard, though: It's easy to tell when someone looks ill at ease in their clothing and just can't "pull it off." If

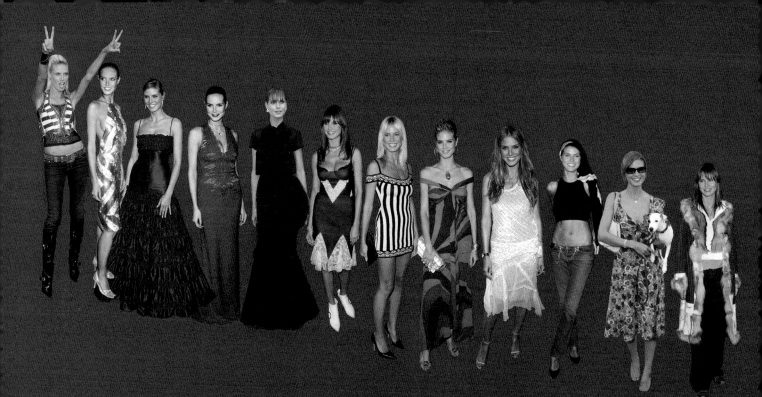

When those bulbs start flashing, you've just got to hope that your clothes fit and you don't trip!

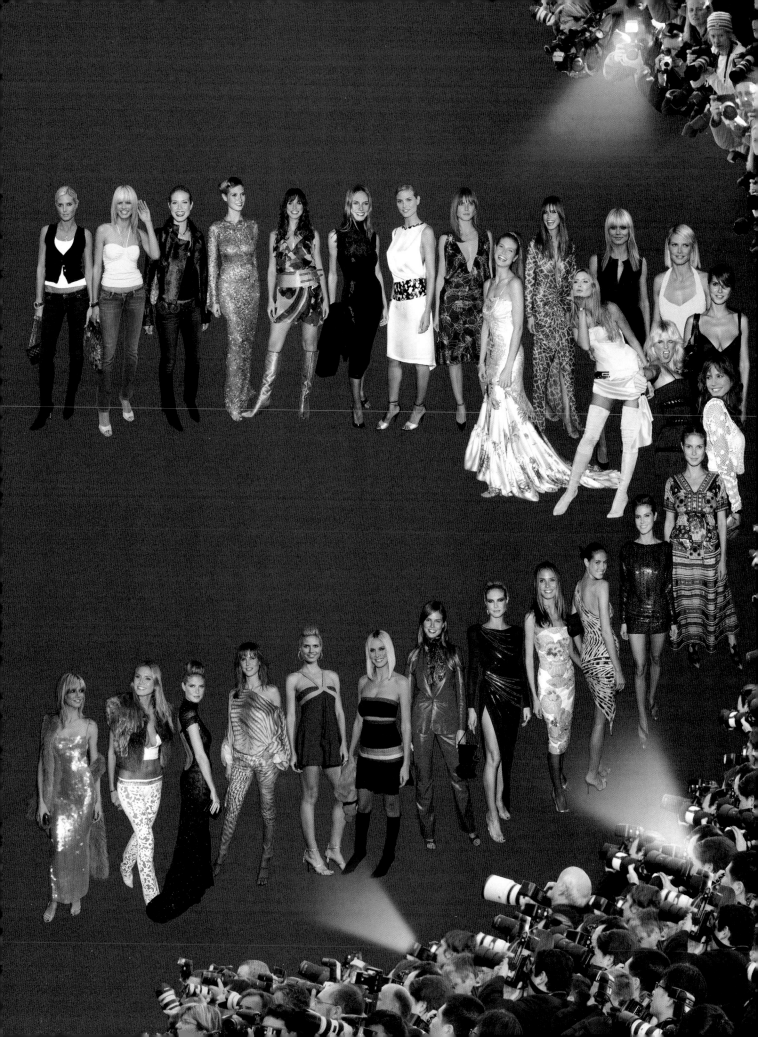

# 10 STEPS FROM RUNWAY TO *YOUR* WAY
BY FASHION STYLIST RACHEL ZOE ROSENZWEIG

*When I met Rachel, an L.A.-based fashion stylist, I was in dire need of a wardrobe overhaul. I always love the out-fits she chooses for me—and she's helped me develop my own sense of style. Here are her insights that can work for anyone.*

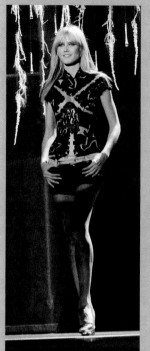

You don't have to have money to have style. Some of the most stylish people I know don't even have a working dishwasher, while the woman who walks into Gucci and buys whatever she wants may be incapable of putting a look together on her own. This alone should lower the intimidation factor when it comes to fashion.

**1. ADMIT YOU NEED HELP.** It's impossible to change if you don't come to terms with your stylistic shortcomings. It's something I have to gently suggest to clients; you can take cues from candid friends and colleagues. ("You look so nice today!" or "Red is a good color for you.")

**2. DON'T COPY THE RUNWAYS; INTERPRET THEM.** If you just mimic a certain look, you won't look like *you,* and everyone will notice your discomfort. Also, almost no one who follows fashion clones a look head to toe; you want to mix up complementary ideas from different designers.

**3. CLIP AND SAVE.** To help you find new ideas, clip pictures from magazines and cata-logs that you really like, put them together, and see what emerges. Are there pieces with similar patterns? Colors? Cuts? Are you gravitating toward skirts worn with boots? Colors that pop more brightly than what's typical in your closet? Certain combinations of accessories? Also watch fashion TV shows on channels like E! and the Style Network for inspiration.

**4. DON'T BE A FASHION VICTIM.** Each season there are several dominant trends, but you don't have to embrace them all at once. Pick one that works for you.

**5. GET A PRO.** If you can't afford a stylist, you can hire a personal shopper at some major department stores at lit-tle or no extra cost. Or, on your next shopping expedition, bring a friend you trust for her brutal candor.

**6. QUALITY OVER QUANTITY.** For classics, it's better to save up for one designer coat or pair of black wool pants than it is to stock up on lots of less expensive outfits. In the end, you'll spend about the same amount; with the lat-ter strategy, though, the clothes will fall apart far more quickly and you'll be left with stuff that will be "out" in months or less.

**7. FIND CHEAP TRENDY PIECES.** On the other hand, for this season's most ephemeral looks, hit discount places like H&M, Express, and Gap, which knock off fashion trends so quickly you can find almost any current look.

**8. OLD IS NEW.** Go vintage (like so many Hollywood starlets) and spend next to nothing on classic designs and designers.

**9. CUSTOMIZE IT.** Bring a picture you like to your local tailor. I know a cash-challenged assistant in the fashion industry who wanted to wear a Christian Dior dress she'd seen in a magazine, so she bought some less expensive fab-ric, went to the tailor, and got what she wanted—for $250, not $2,500.

**10. HAVE FUN.** Not every look you put together will be a winner. But you won't know until you try, will you?

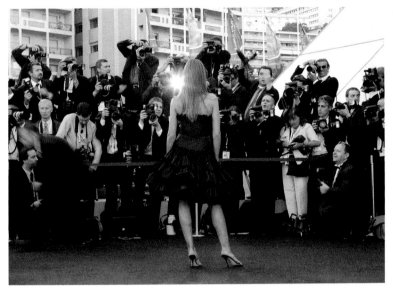

you've ever seen an obviously eccentric character trapped in a corporate uniform, you know what I mean.)

It can also be an expensive way of expressing yourself, so take advantage of what you have and what you already know works for you. On the flip side, don't be afraid to branch out, even if it's just a little at first, from your norm. The first few times you try to be different or experimental, it may be scary. I have professionals helping me achieve different looks, but friends are invaluable resources when a personal stylist's not around. Ask for opinions! I do. I ask trusted friends all the time—"Is this too much?" . . . "What if I wear it like this?"

But, I confess, sometimes I take the advice and sometimes I don't. Because with fashion, it can be bolder to go for it even if you're told the other outfit is more appropriate. Who cares?! I go with my gut instinct. It's almost always right—except on rare occasions. Once I got myself into a predicament when I cajoled my friend, designer Roberto Cavalli, to cut an extremely expensive leather embroidered dress for me to wear to an awards show (after his design office had emphatically told me "no way," I just called him in Italy myself!). Well, let's just say it got cut a little *too* short—it didn't look great, and I felt uncomfortable, so I went with something else. Don't worry, I made up for it by wearing Cavalli often (though not exactly that one —may the poor leather dress RIP) and mentioning his name lots and *lots* of times.

So give yourself a break, permission to change your mind, just like I often do right before I leave the house. That's a girl's (and a guy's) prerogative. Go with what feels right at a given moment. And, hey, if it doesn't pan out and you (okay, I) end up on a worst-dressed list, laugh, shrug, and go about your day. New day, new outfit—easy.

Although I've spent the last few paragraphs encouraging you to make a fashion statement, sometimes you want the statement to be an *under*statement. When choosing a wardrobe, consider the context: If I'm attending a charity event, I'm not going to proudly display my cleavage; for a business meeting, I'll wear black pants and heels and take the prestige bag rather than the everyday bag. Predictable as it may be, I'll feel more comfortable in a (nonstodgy) suit than some slinky or slouchy number, and for that reason I'll be more likely to get my message across, and they'll take it, and me, seriously. It's pretty funny sometimes to see people's disappointed reactions, but honestly, what do they expect me to show up in for a serious meeting—a bikini?!

# make it personal

When I travel I'm always on the lookout for something unique and cool and very me, that thing that could set a little trend by itself (maybe!): a great funky studded belt from Las Vegas, just this side of tacky, or a vintage Stones tee from the Paris flea market, or a one-of-a-kind necklace from Attilio Codignato in Venice, which specializes in very old jewelry pieces with interesting histories.

Even though access and money get you a very nice wardrobe, nothing's more satisfying than scoring something

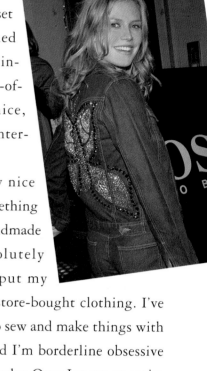

original or handmade that you absolutely adore. I also put my own twist on store-bought clothing. I've always loved to sew and make things with my hands—and I'm borderline obsessive about my Bedazzler. Once I spent an entire flight between New York and London studding the back of a denim jacket with hundreds of Swarovski crystals—my own take on rocker-chick chic. For a recent TV promo for my stint hosting "Shark Week" on the Discovery Channel, I cut out the silk-screened portion of a *Jaws* T-shirt and studded it by hand onto a tight white tee. Everyone wanted to know where I'd bought it! (I've had offers to buy my one-of-a-kind creations right off my back.)

Some people are born with style, others achieve it (and still others—*hello!*—have it thrust upon them). No matter how you get it, your personal style should express who you are, and help you project who it is you want to be in life. It's easy to dismiss dressing well as the exclusive dominion of

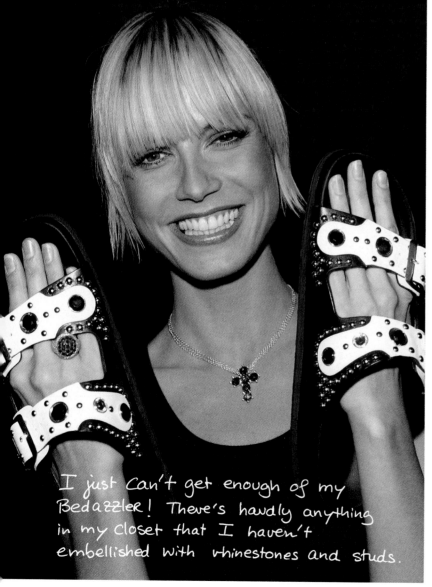

*I just can't get enough of my Bedazzler! There's hardly anything in my closet that I haven't embellished with rhinestones and studs.*

fashion snobs, but a well-honed style sense can not only help you get your foot in the door, but it can also win you the credibility to make you the one with your name on the door.

You know how, when someone says something clever, you think, *Why didn't I say that?* With a little money, not much work, and a good helping of imagination, you'll be making fashion statements bold enough that, when people pass you, they'll be muttering, *Why can't I wear that?*

## FOR GUYS: LINGERIE-BUYING 101

*Only the rarest sugar daddy can afford a diamond-studded bra and panties, but any kind of underwear makes a great gift—if you're sending the right message.*

**1.** Unsure about her size? Err on the small side. Don't insult her with some XL negligee when you can flatter her with a medium (max!).

**2.** Use the saleswomen for advice. They've seen and heard everything from men about what their mates are like in their most private moments—some of which is unprintable here!

**3.** Buy items in the style you think most suits her, not the ones you've always admired in laddie magazines. If she's got a drawerful of big cotton undies, don't go for racy G-strings with pearls running down the crotch. However, once you've purchased a few pieces you know she'll like, then you can throw in a couple fantasy items. (Call it shopping foreplay.)

**4.** When you present her with your purchase, don't smack your lips like some dog in heat. And don't make her strip on the spot and model it for you. Set a mood for seduction: The lingerie's allure works best when she's a willing participant.

**5.** Reminder: It's for *her.* Don't try it on yourself.

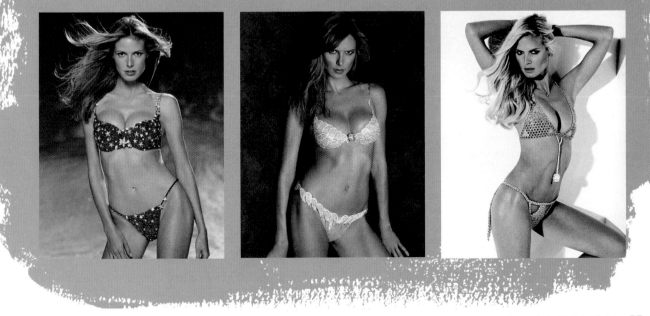

# ORGANIZE YOUR LIFE—OR JUST YOUR CLOSET

BY LINDA ROTHSCHILD, NEW YORK ORGANIZATIONAL GURU AND FOUNDER OF CROSS IT OFF YOUR LIST

*I met Linda after she did a total overhaul of my publicist Desiree's closets. Linda's demanding, high-profile clients love her rigorous sense of order. Here's her advice on how to organize your wardrobe, and just about everything else.*

The purpose of organizing your closet—or any room in your house—should be to arrange it so you can get to things effortlessly and quickly. Many people just keep buying the same articles of clothing because they forget they already own them, or have no idea where they are. Out of sight, out of mind.

Organizing is something you should do all the time. You can do one big purge yearly, if not seasonally, but it is not simply about getting rid of things—it's about having access to what you want and storing everything so you can find it.

**1. STAND IN YOUR CLOSET AND REMOVE EVERYTHING, ONE ITEM AT A TIME.** As you touch each piece of clothing, ask yourself some really honest questions: Do I wear this? Do I really love it? Does it irritate my skin every time I put it on? Do these shoes hurt my feet so much I will never wear them again? Have I stopped wearing this, yet can't get rid of it because I blew an entire paycheck on it? Just let it go. Sort into piles for keeping, donating, repairing, or tossing.

**2. THINK INSIDE THE BOX.** I don't strictly adhere to the if-you-haven't-worn-it-in-a-year-then-toss-it rule. Some things are classic or vintage and can be held on to for a time. It's what I call "personal recycling." Box and label, then store in an out-of-the-way place—on a shelf in the closet, or in the attic.

**3. MAXIMIZE SPACE.** Now that everything is out of the closet, figure out how to put it all back in an organized way. Start with the hanging clothes, and organize by type—tops, skirts, pants, jackets, suits. Hang long things with long, short with short. For extra points, organize by color. Figure out what kinds of containers you need to store what you're keeping. Exploit upper and lower spaces: The shelf above the rod is good for stuff you use less often. Use the space underneath your short hanging clothes for shoe boxes or drawers.

**4. BUY GOOD-QUALITY HANGERS.** Wood or plastic, they're not that expensive; they affect how your clothes hang in the closet and, therefore, how they look on you.

**5. LOSE THE DRY-CLEANING BAGS.** They're bad for fabric because they don't breathe or allow the dry-cleaning chemicals to air out. Plus, when you look into your closet and see that sea of plastic, you often miss what's hiding underneath. For infrequently used items, store in canvas bags instead.

**6. GET A FRIEND—ONE YOU TRUST TO BE HONEST—TO HELP YOU EDIT YOUR STUFF.** It's pointless unless she feels comfortable saying, "That's hideous. Throw it out."

**7. FIND A WORTHY PLACE FOR DONATIONS.** If you're struggling to get rid of things you'll never wear again, think about someone who needs them more than you do—could be a friend or your local thrift shop or homeless shelter. Designer duds can go to a resale shop. You may even get a tax deduction.

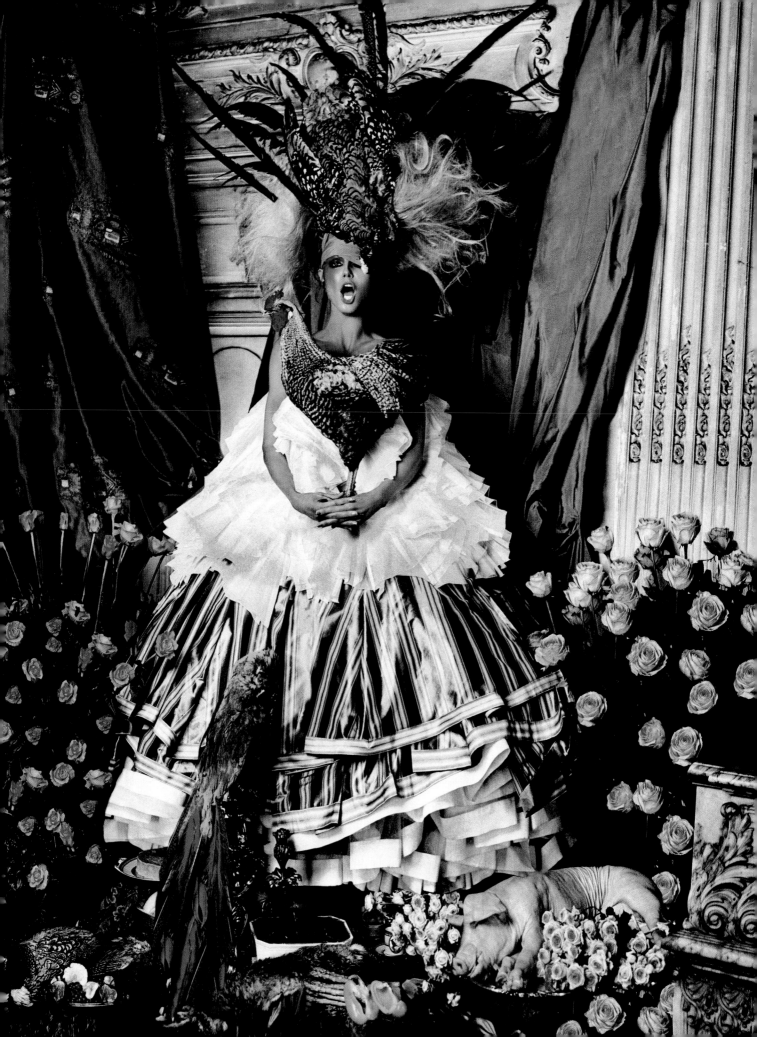

# PHOTOS

*some of my favorites*

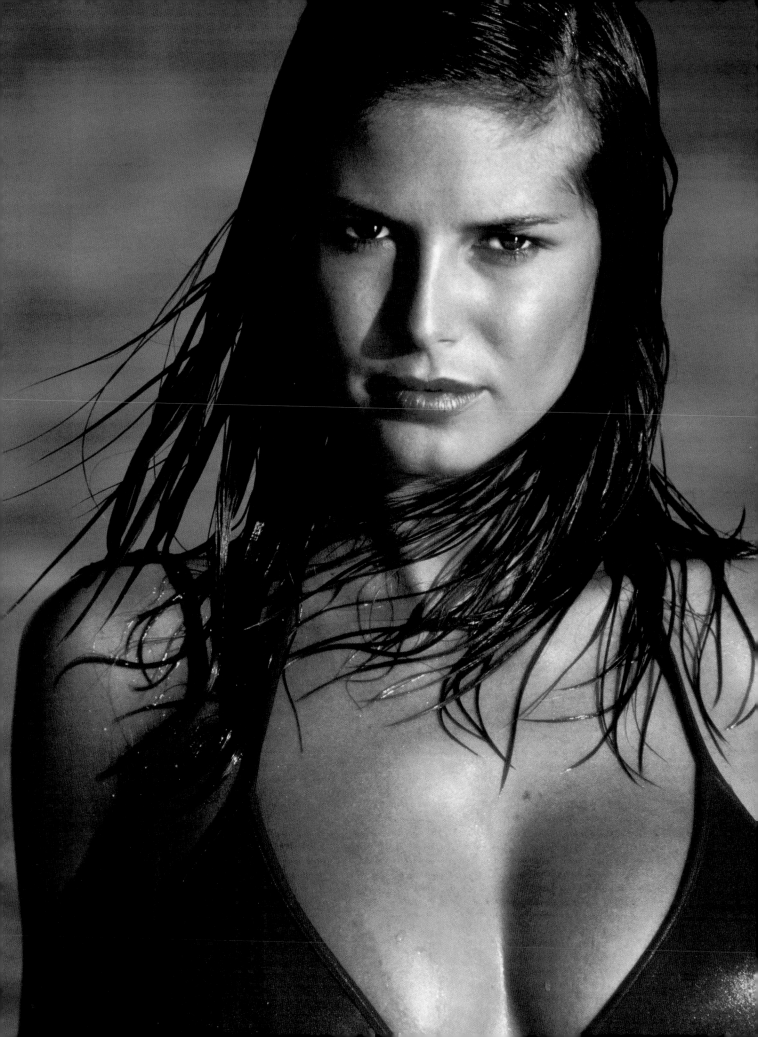

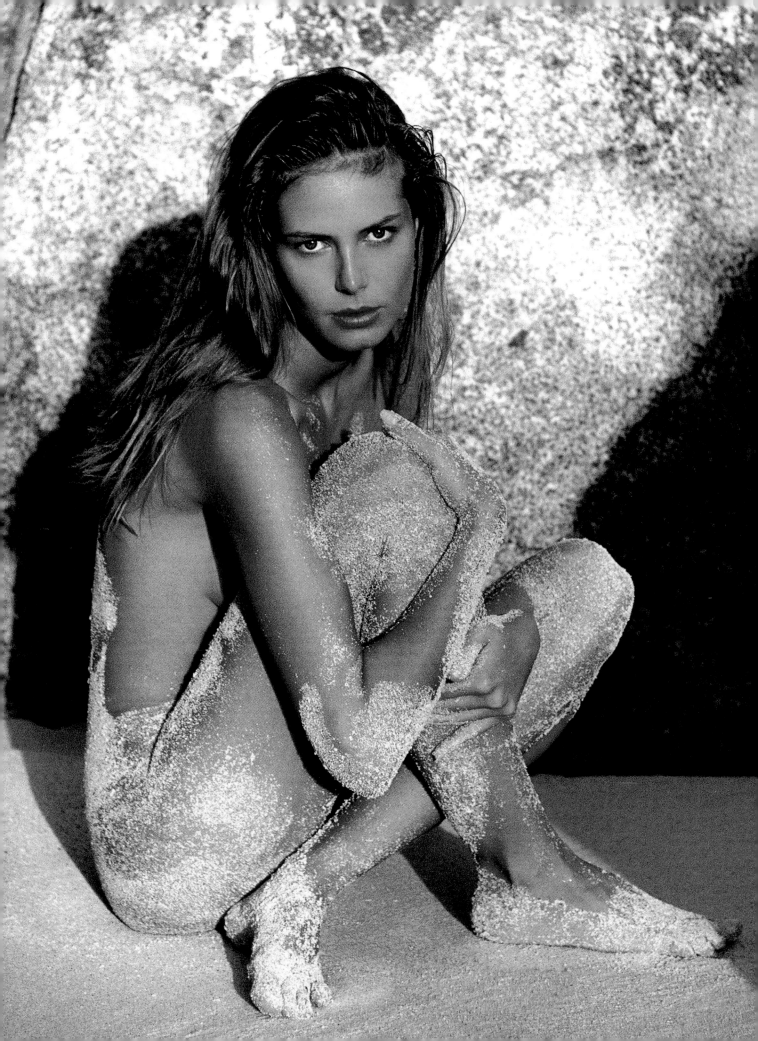

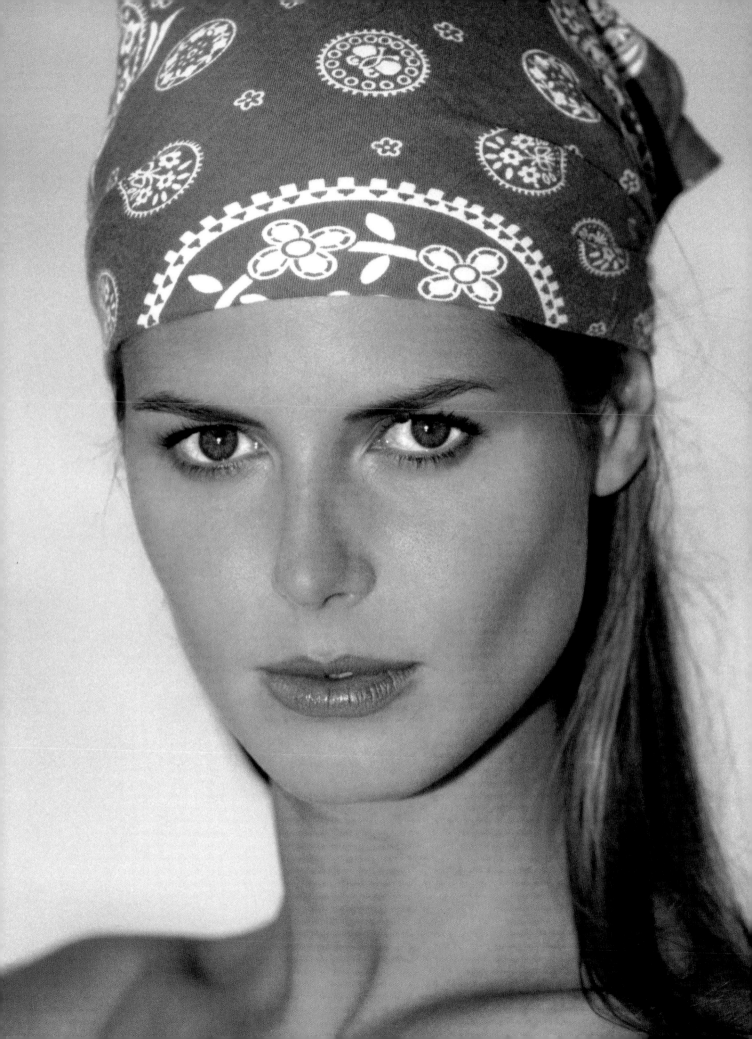

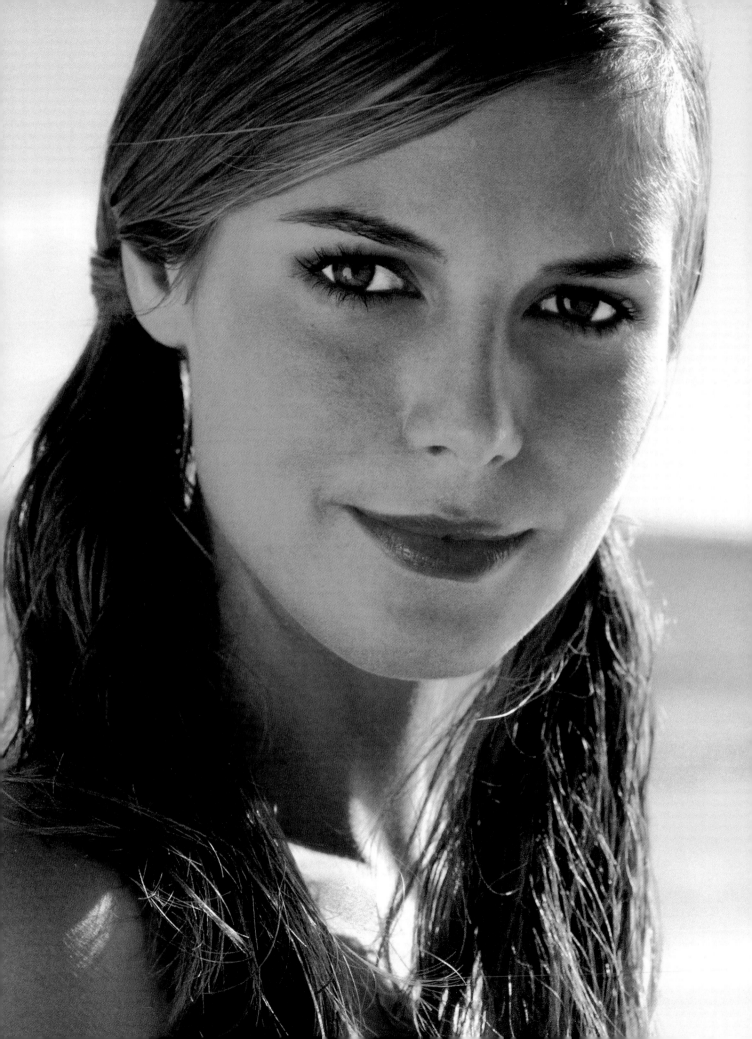

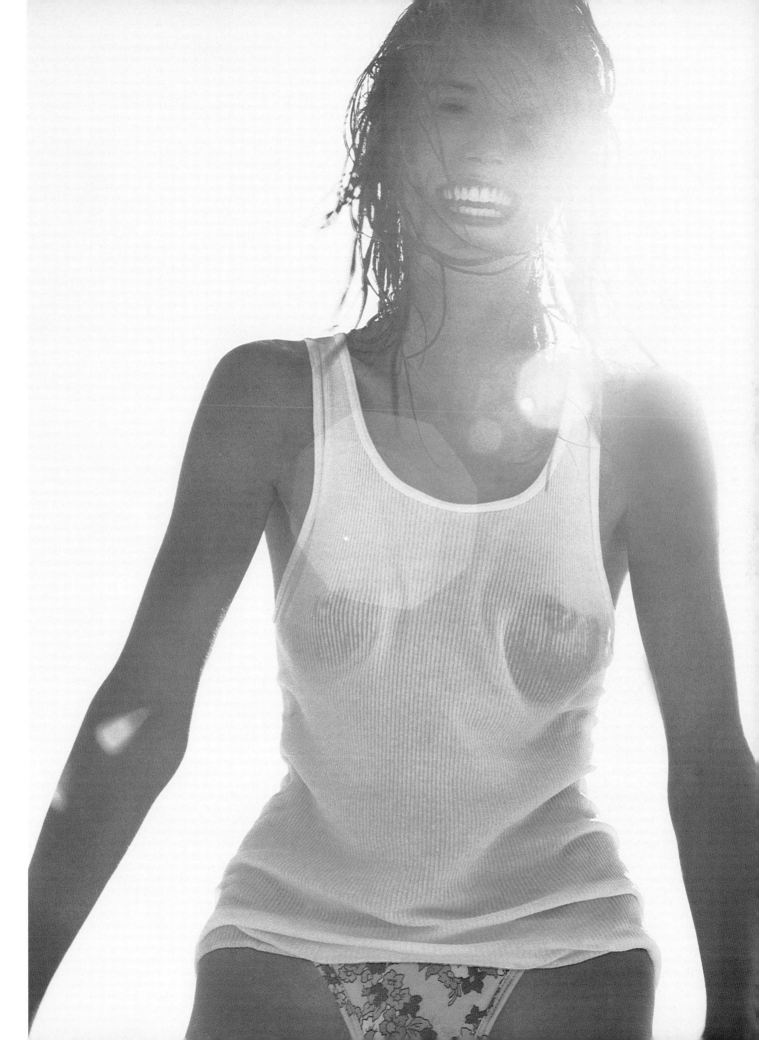

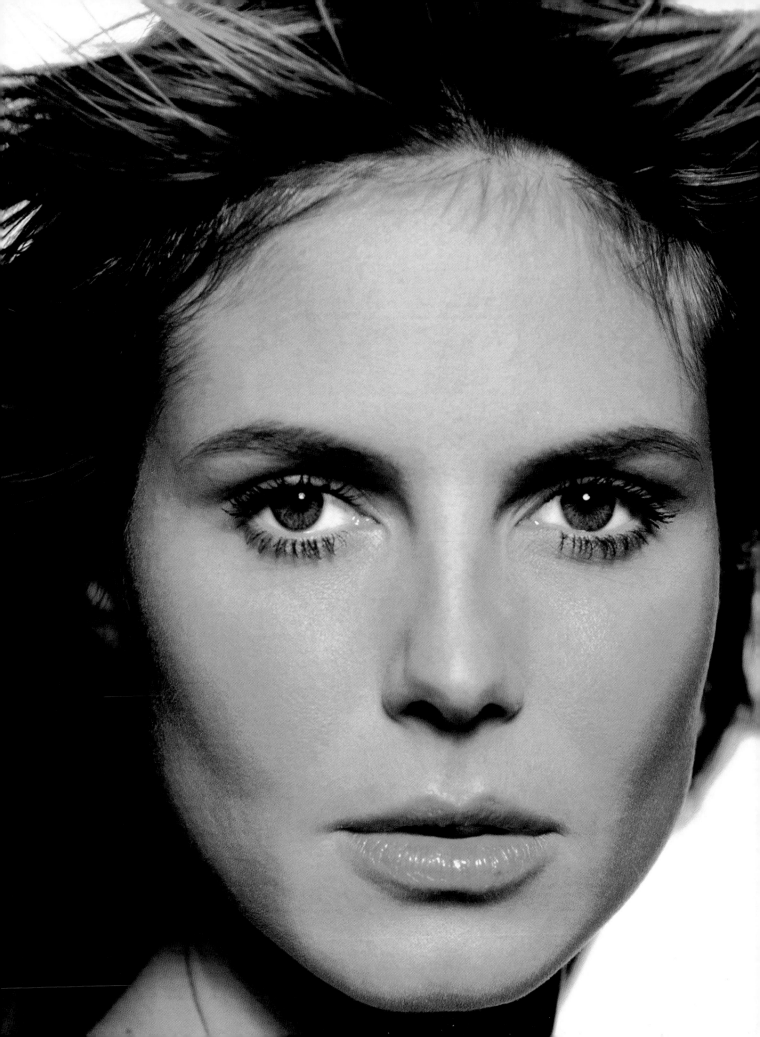

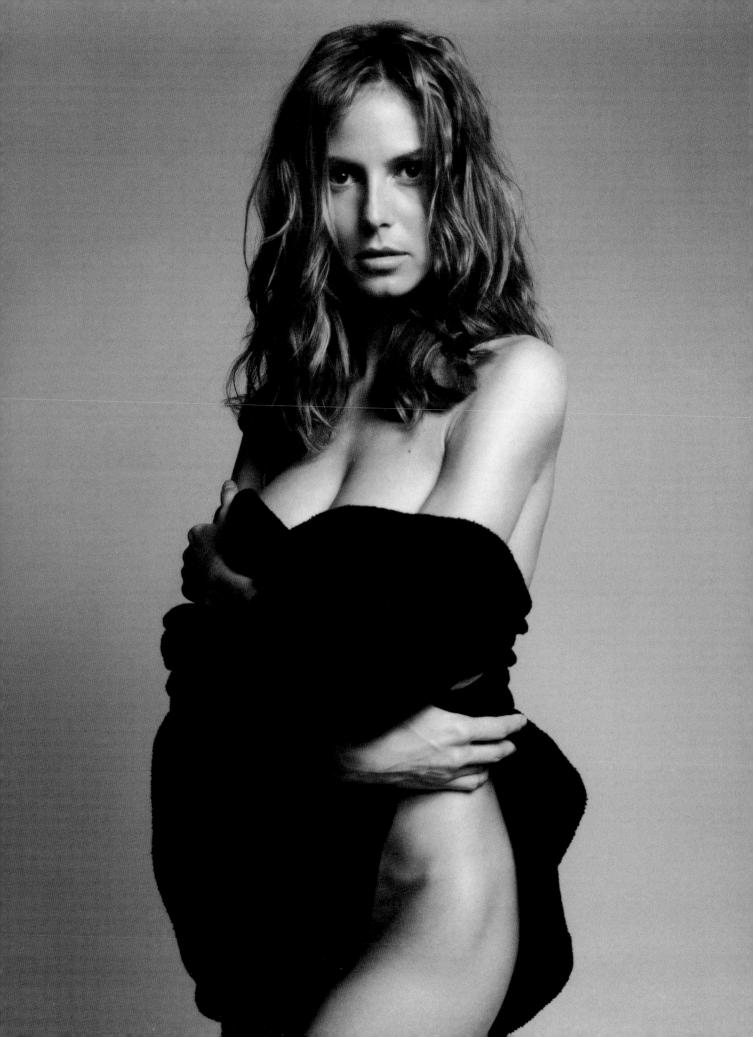

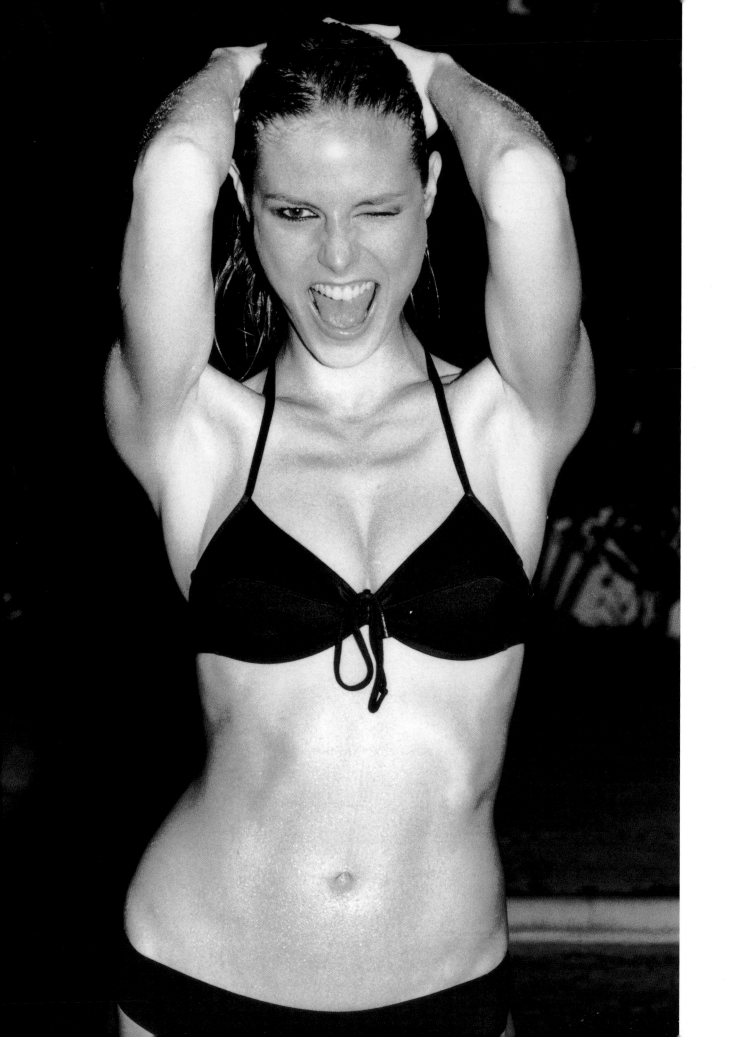

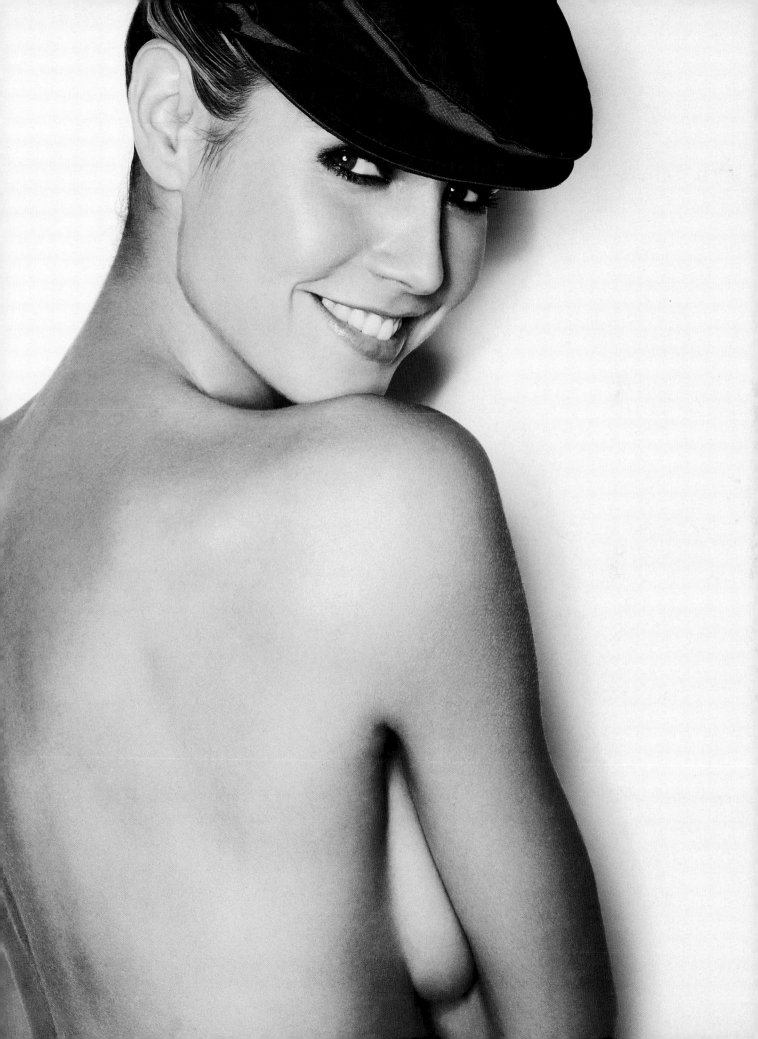

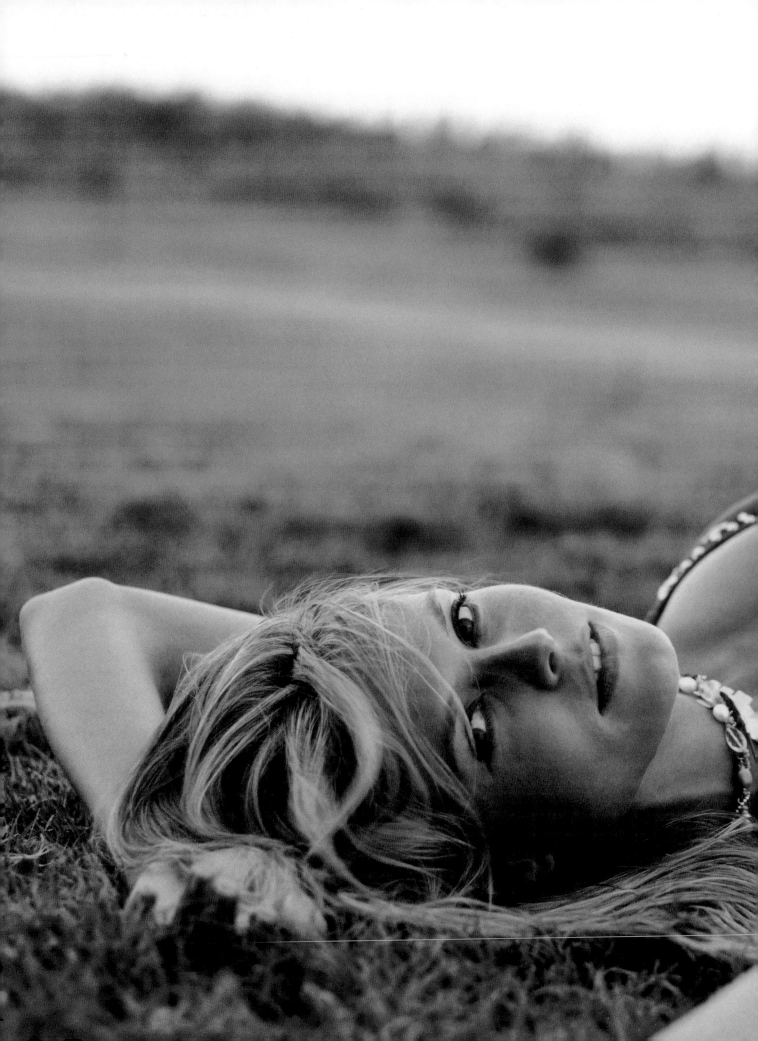

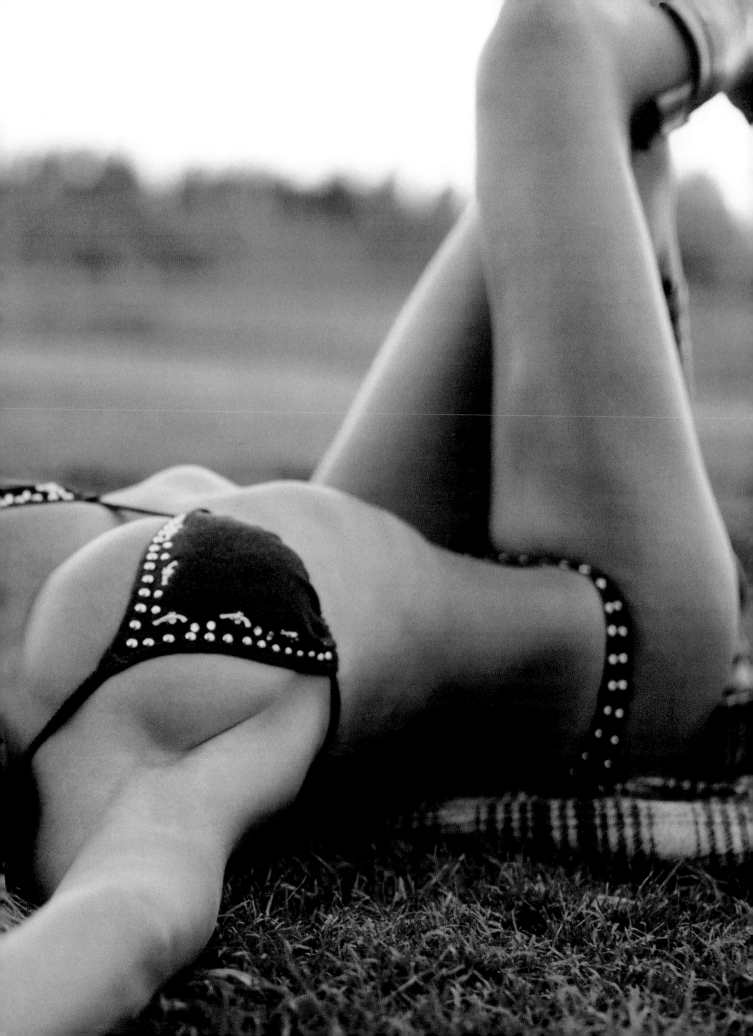

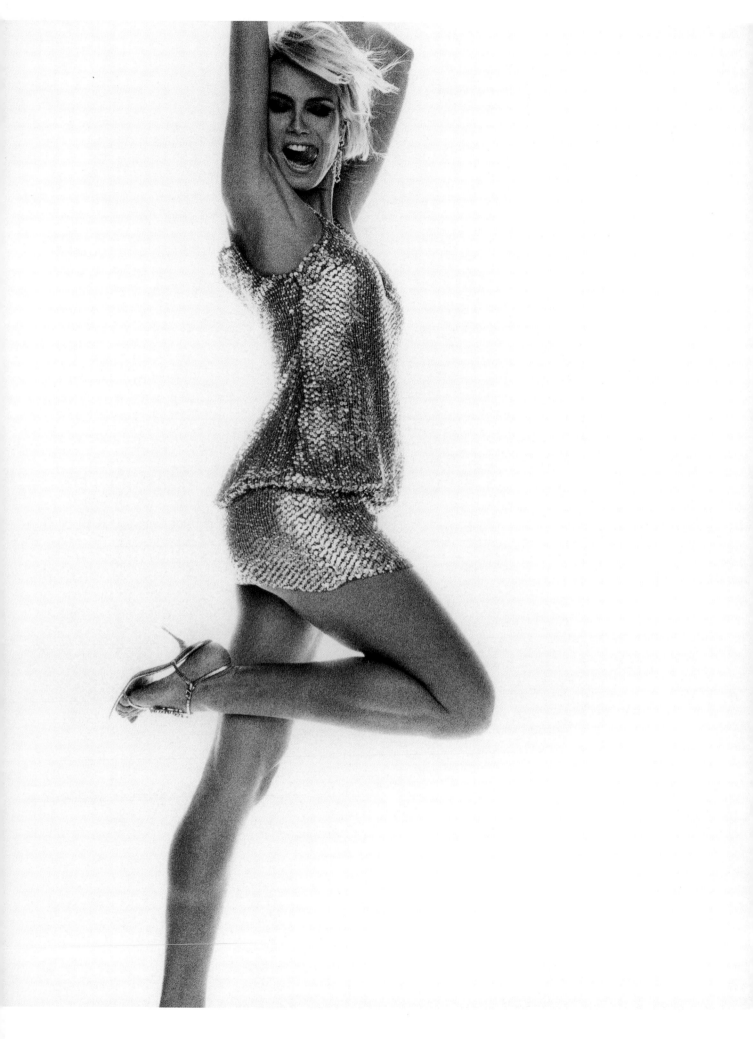

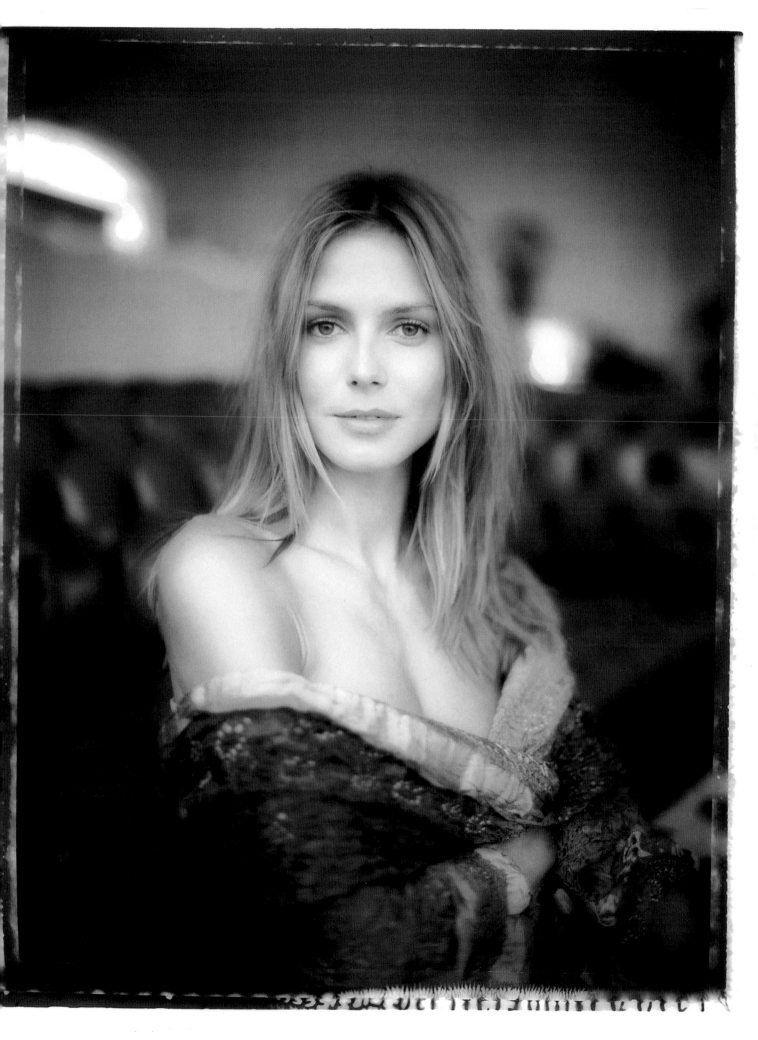

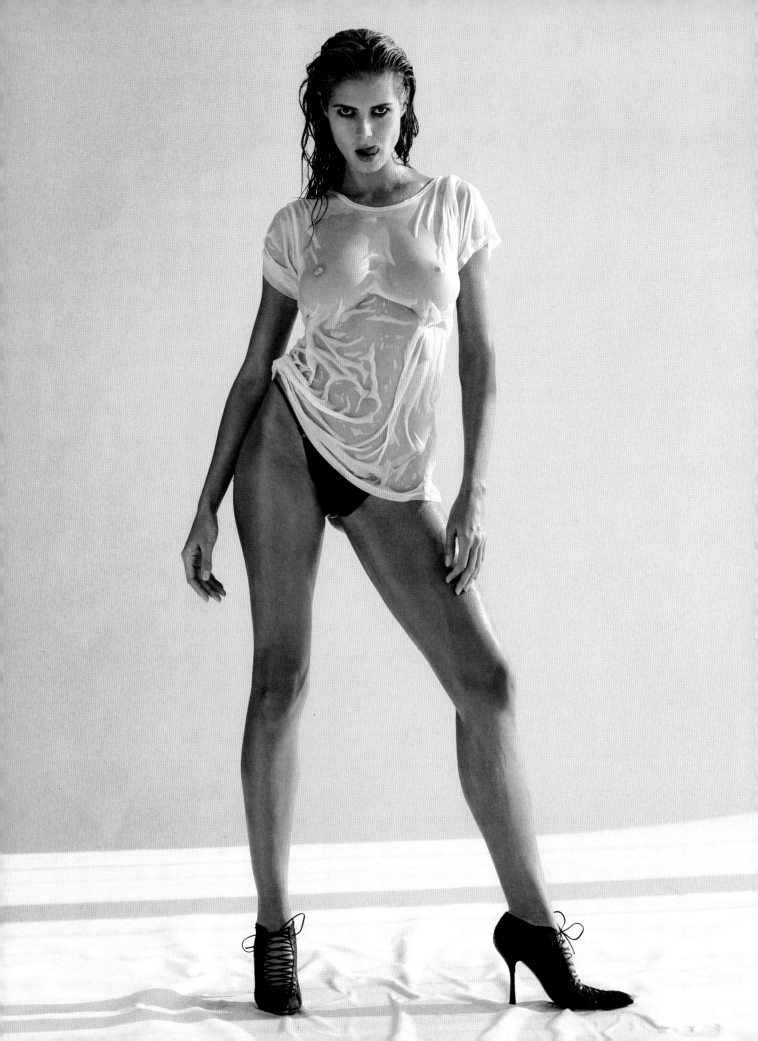

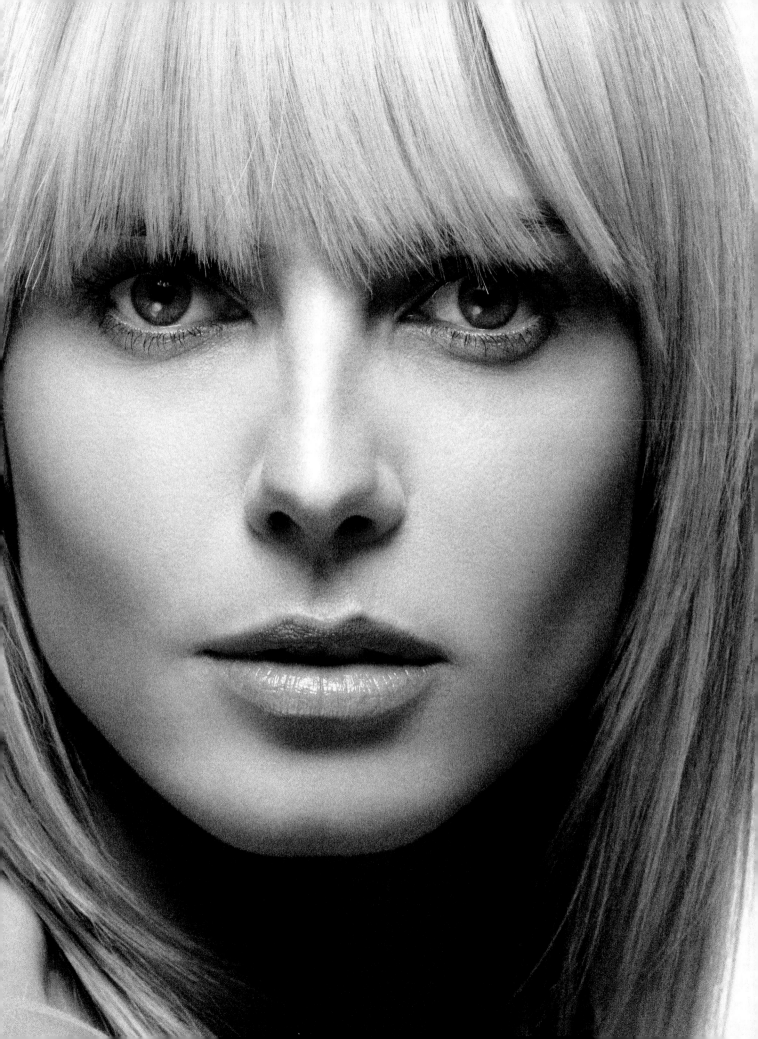

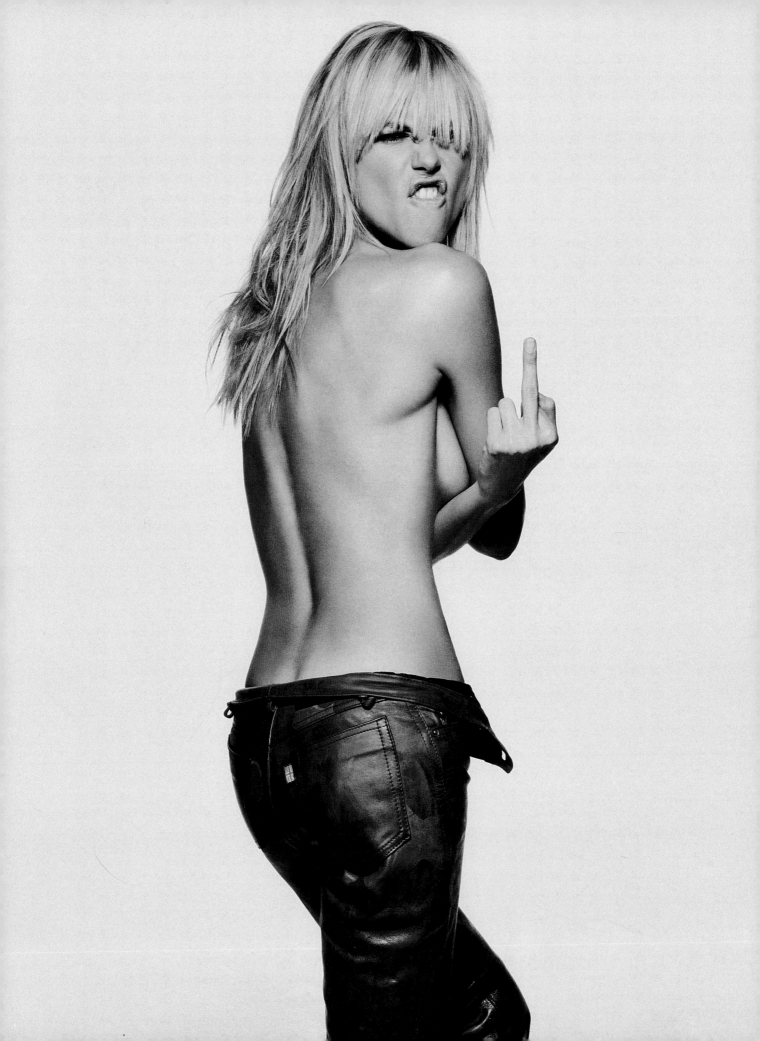

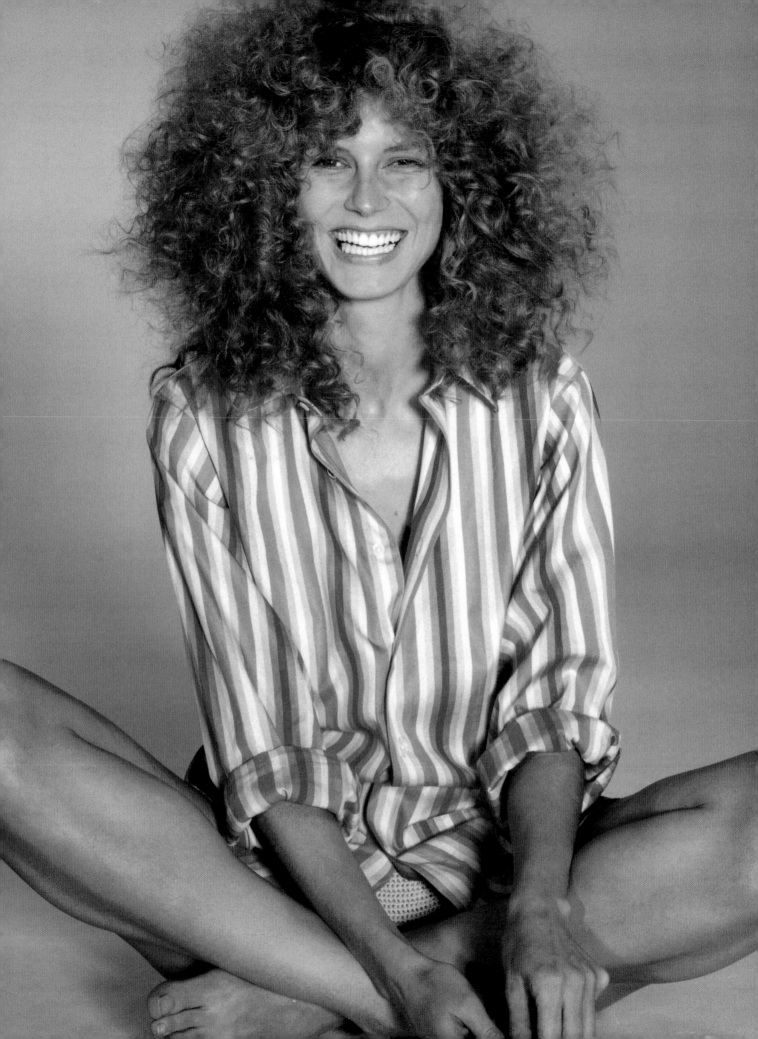

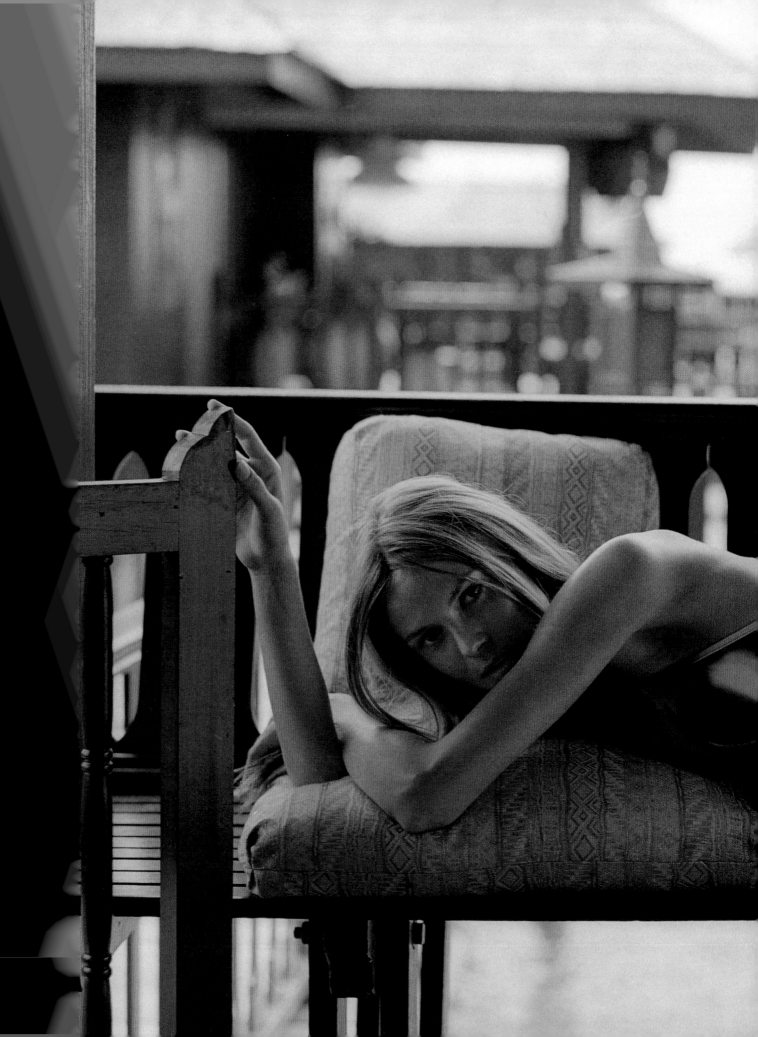

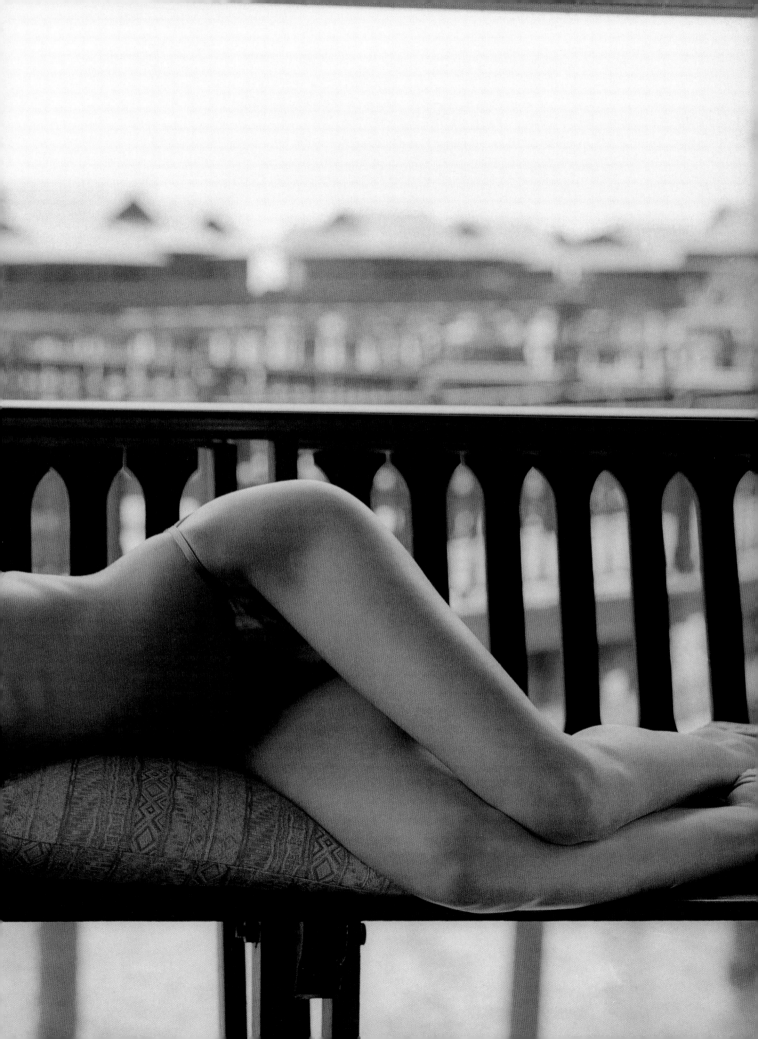

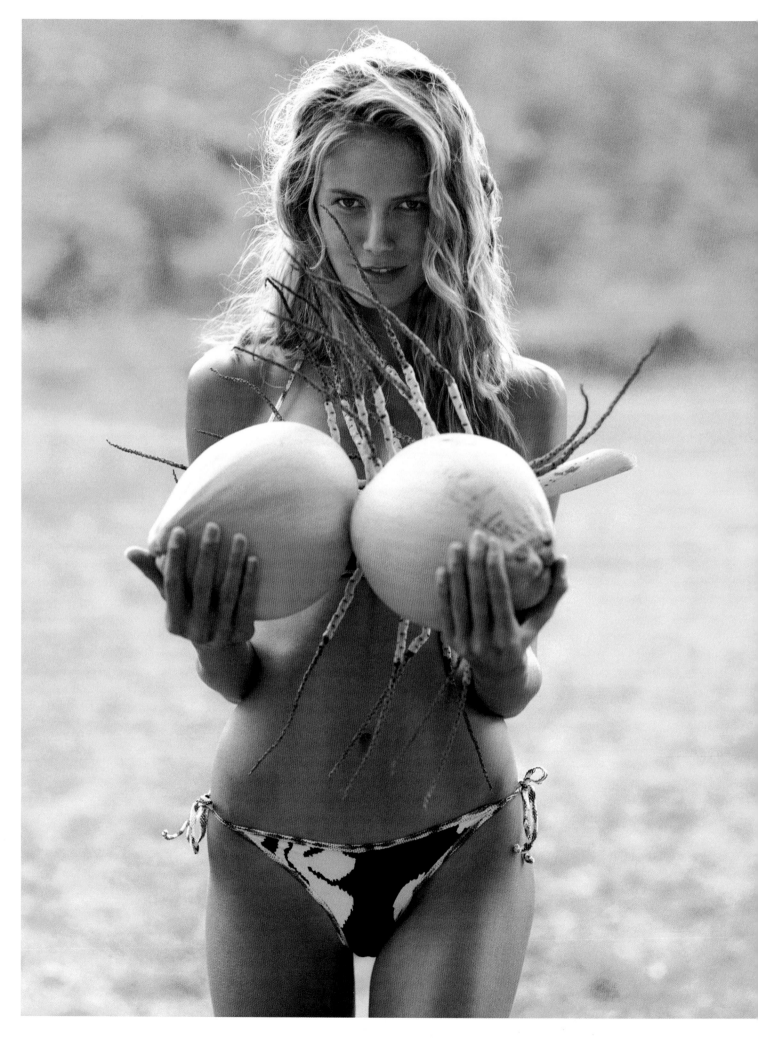

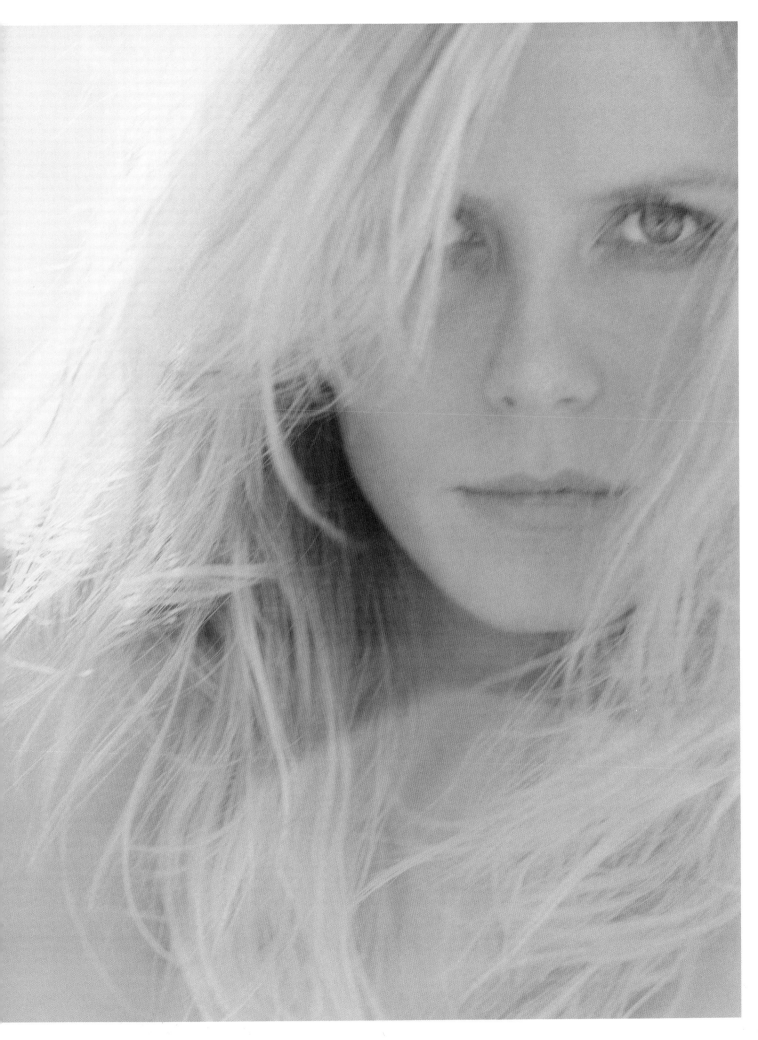

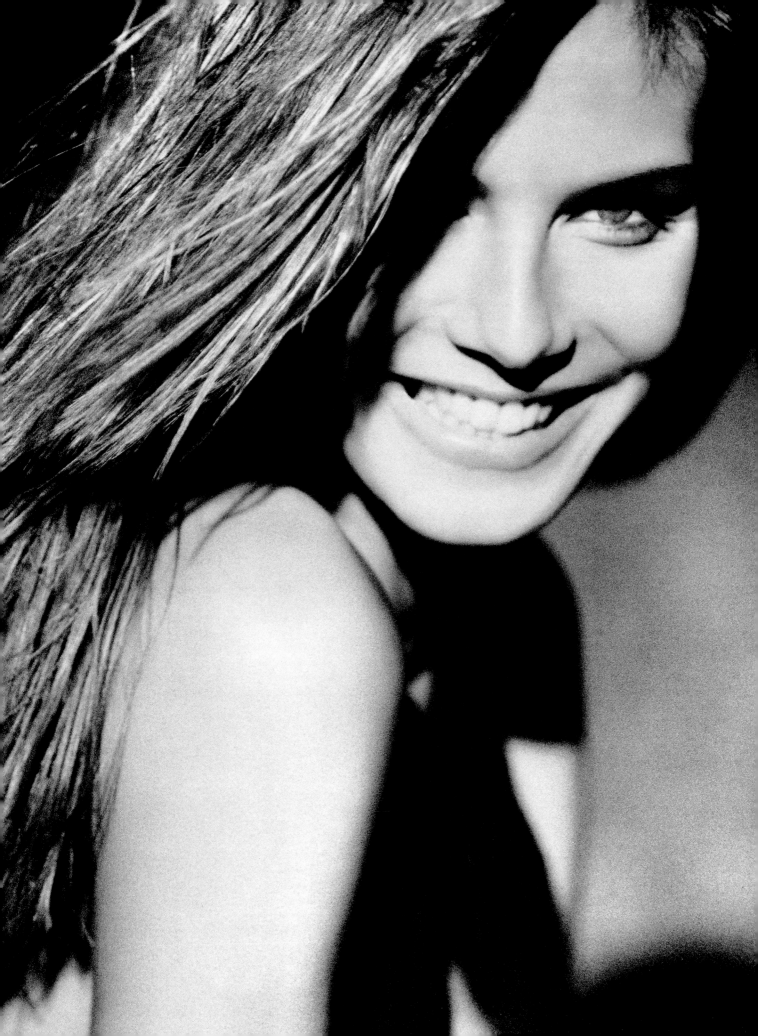

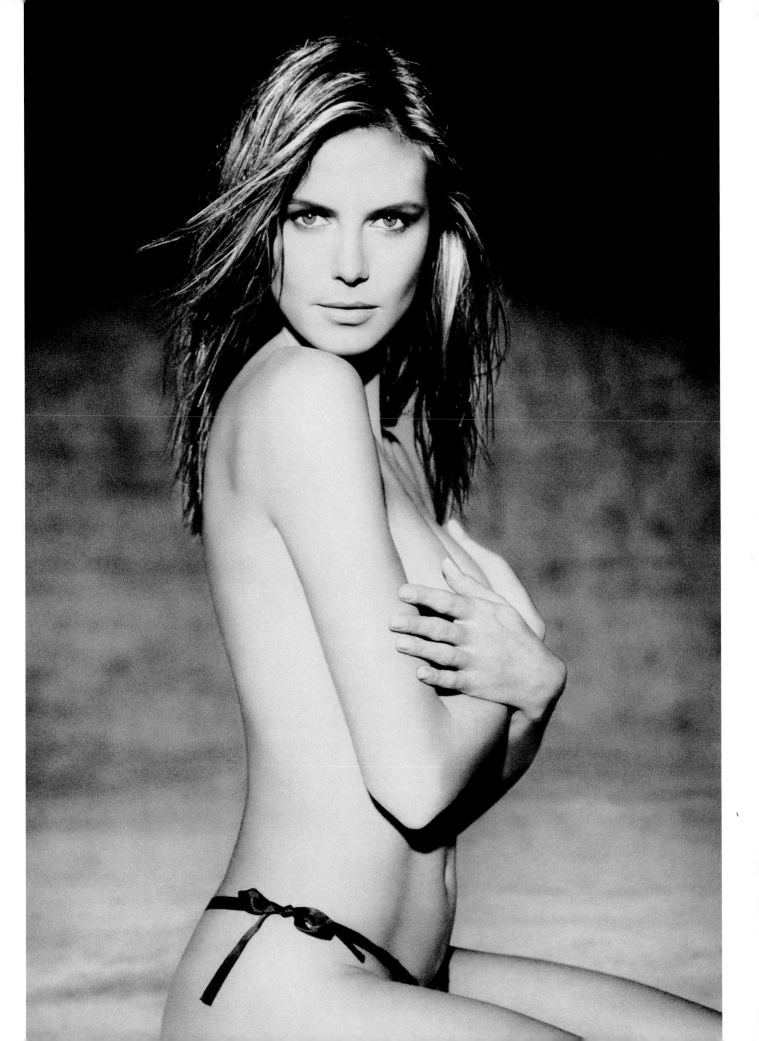

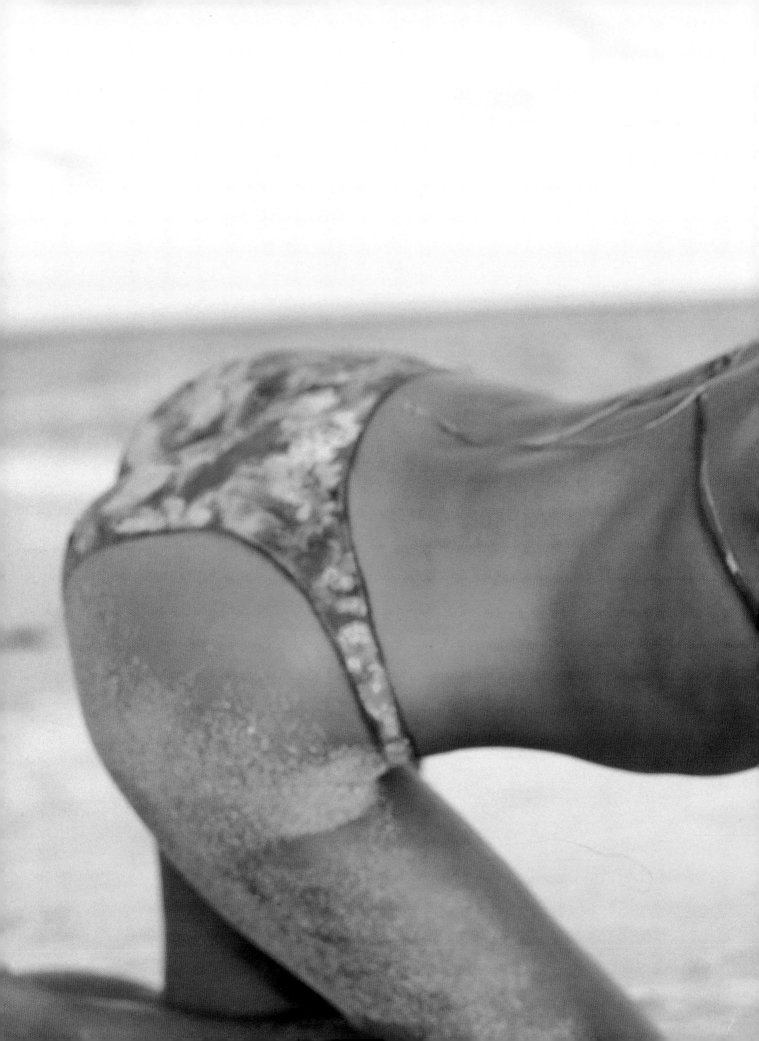

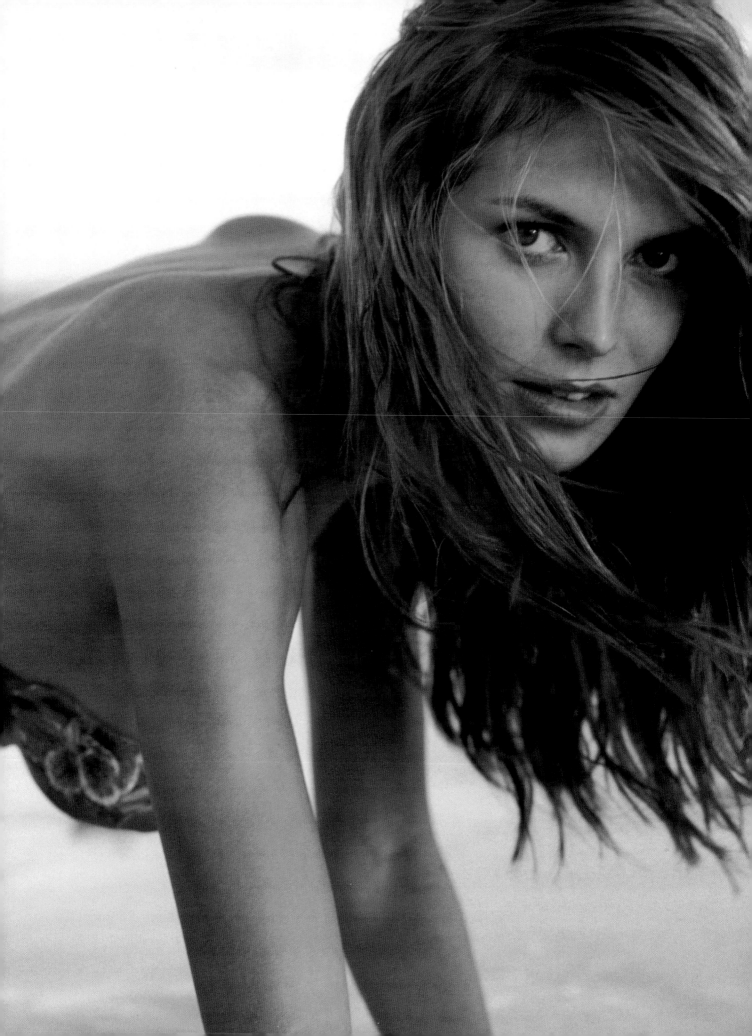

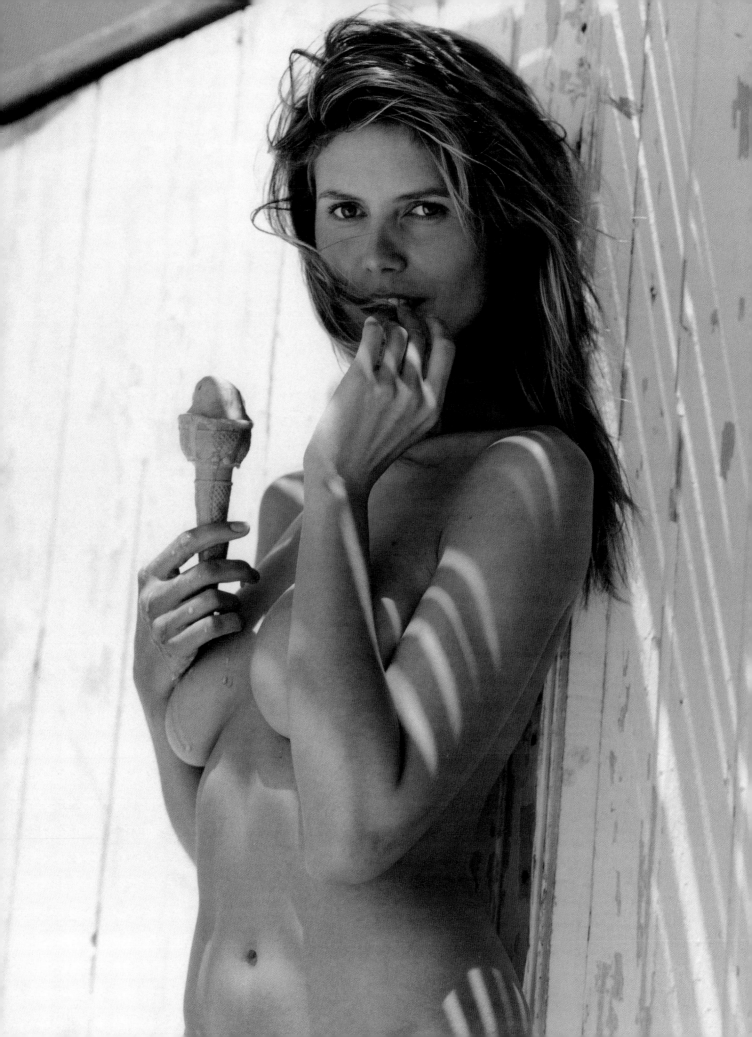

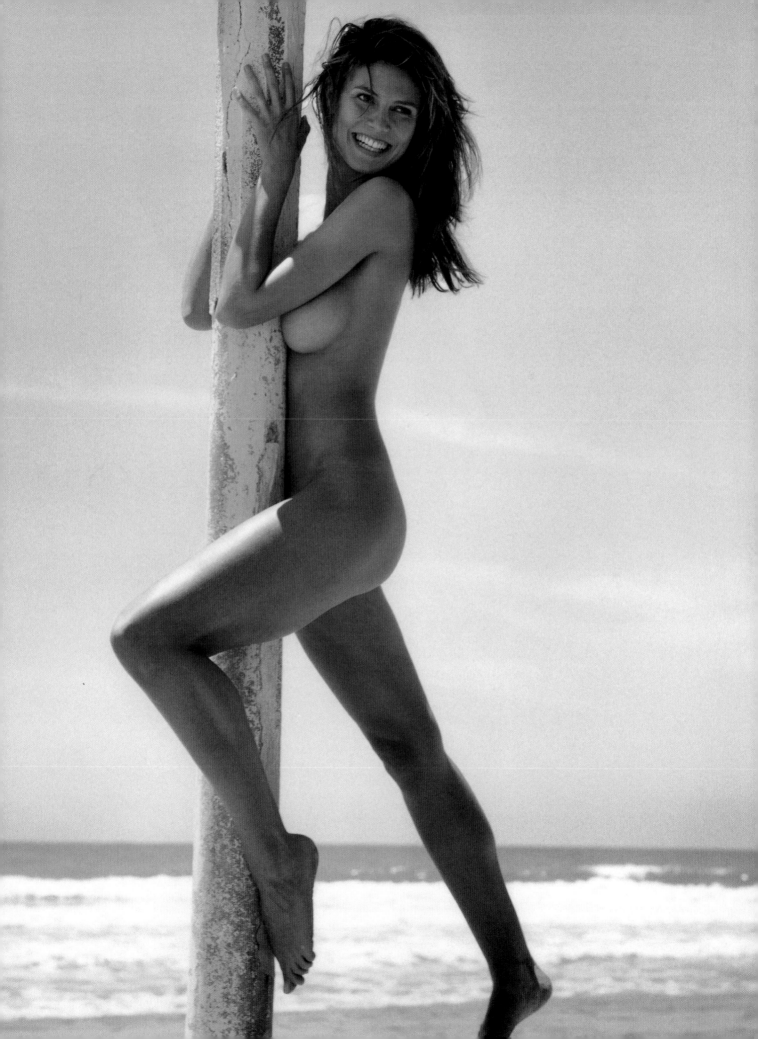

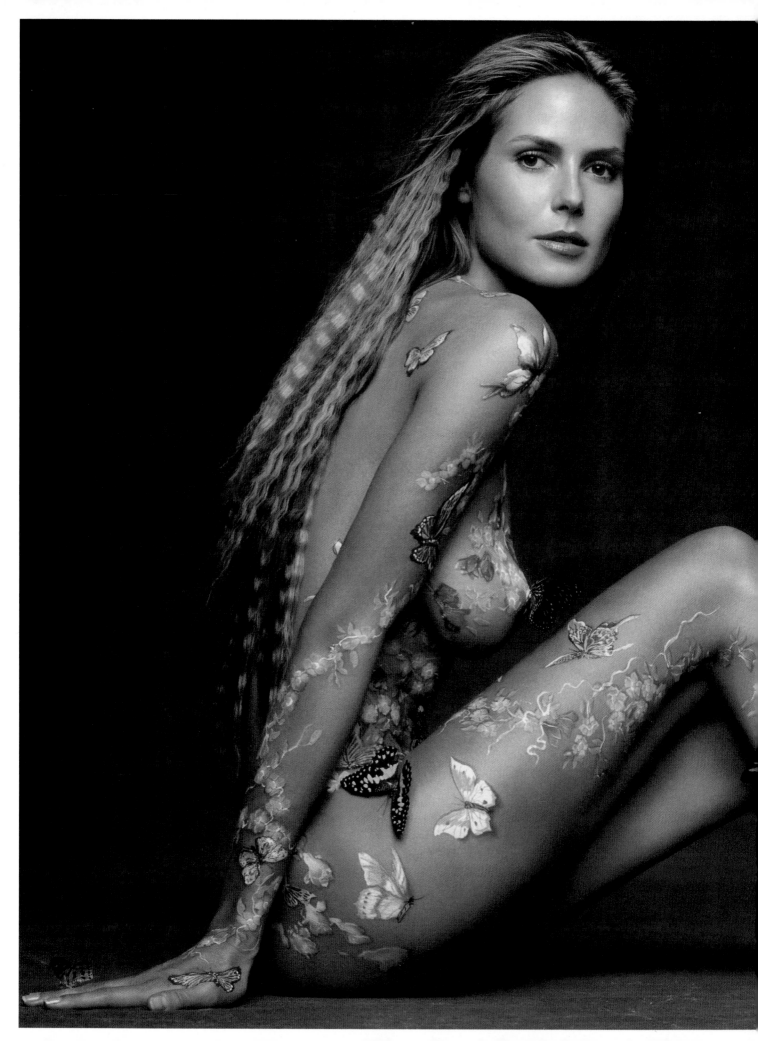

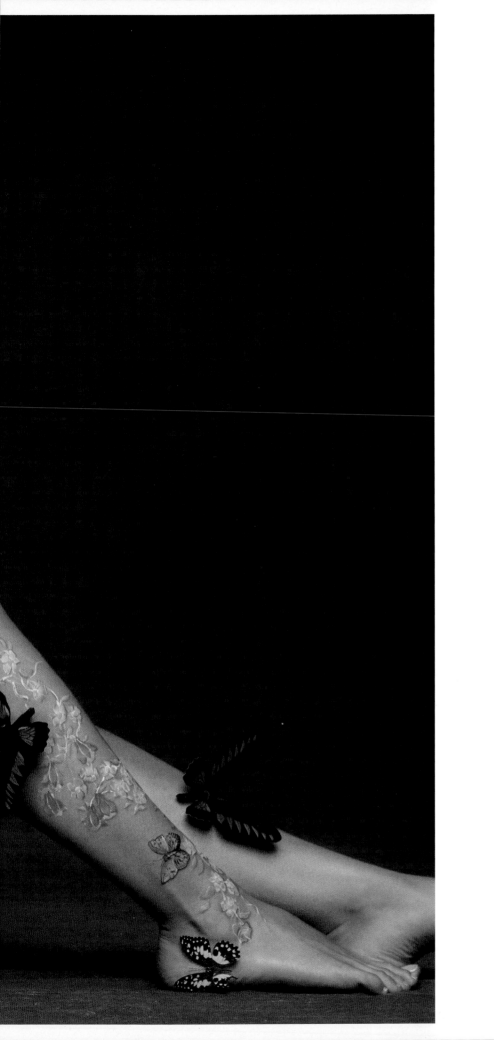

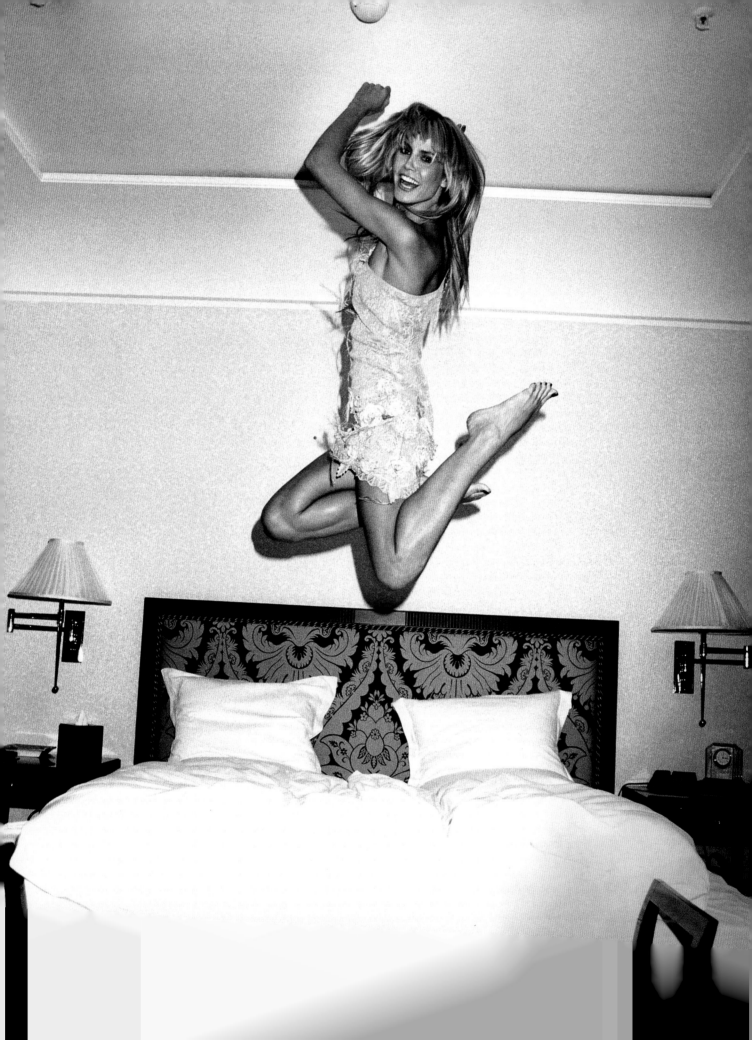

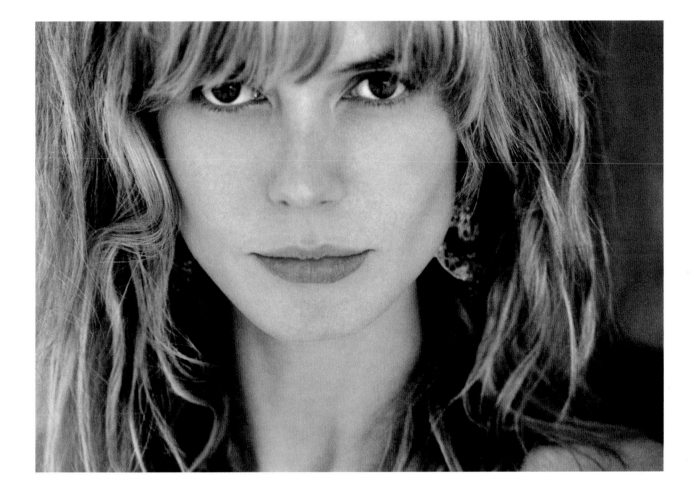

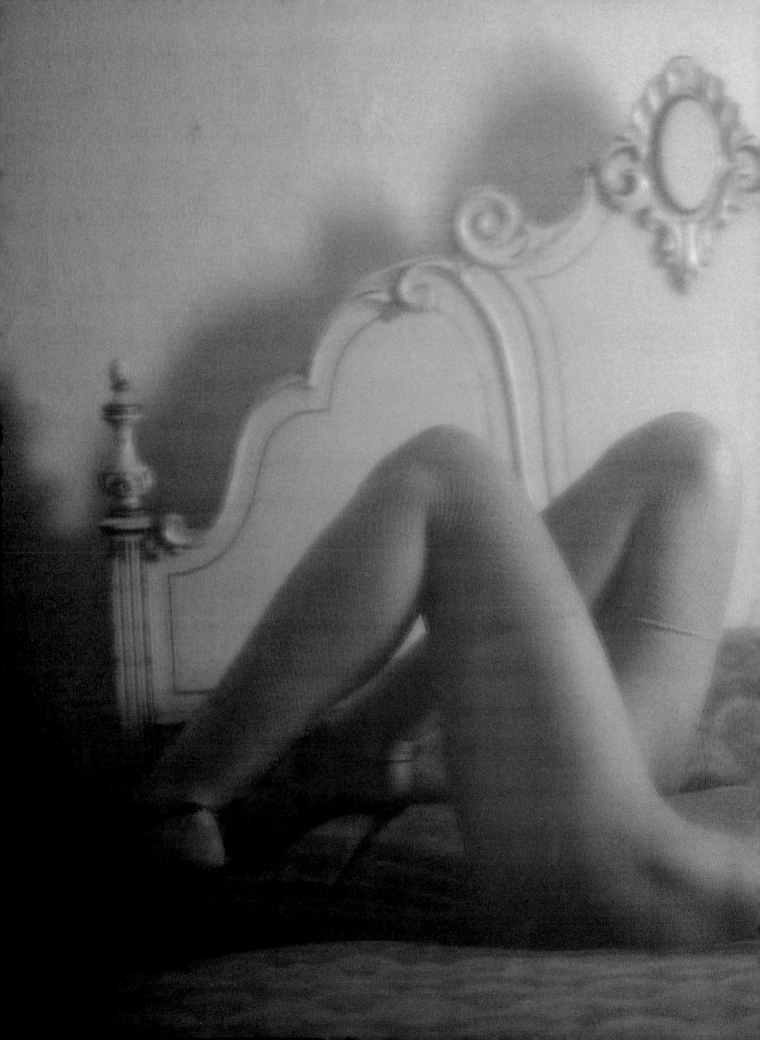

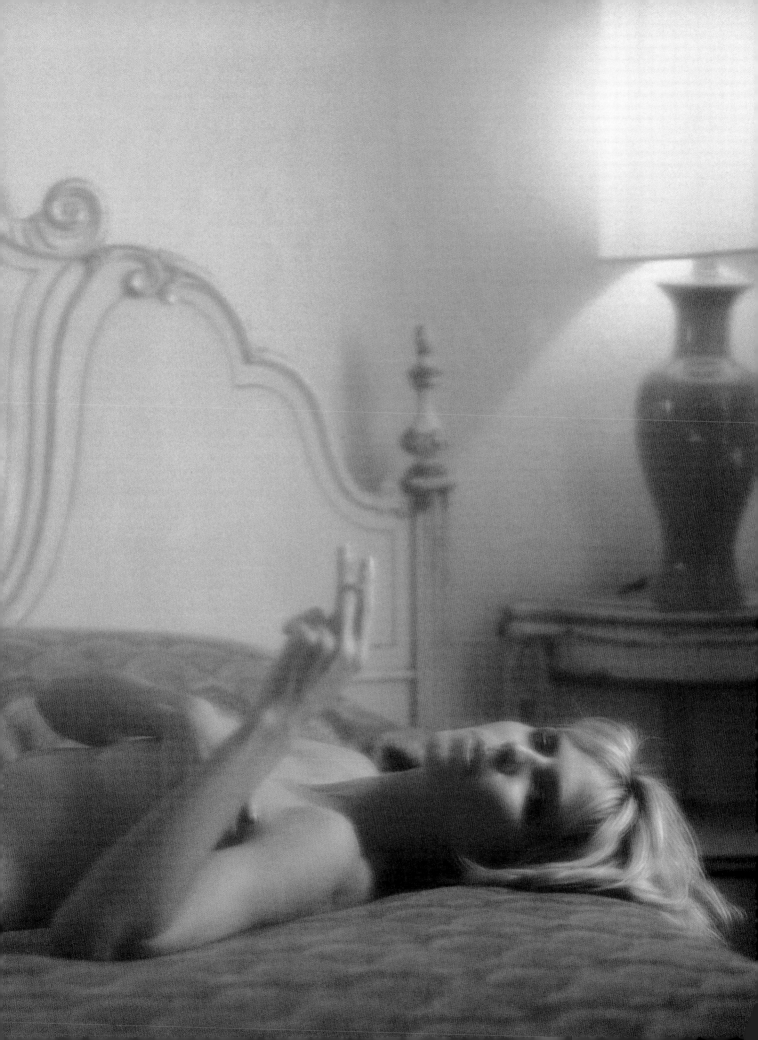

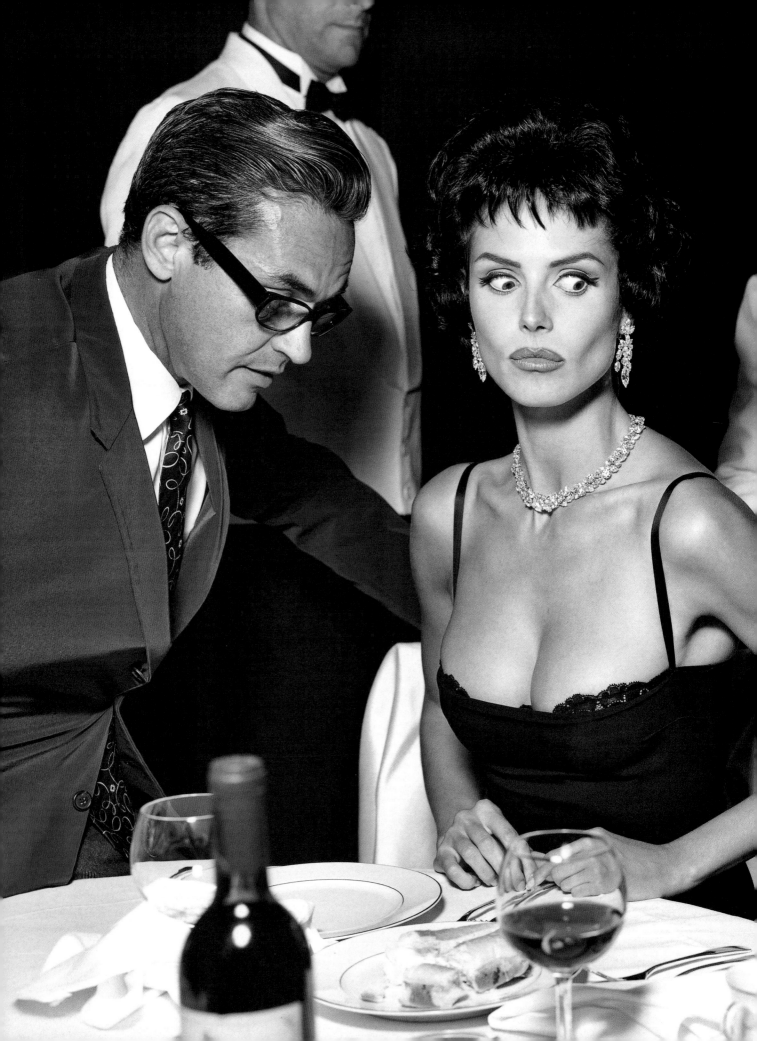

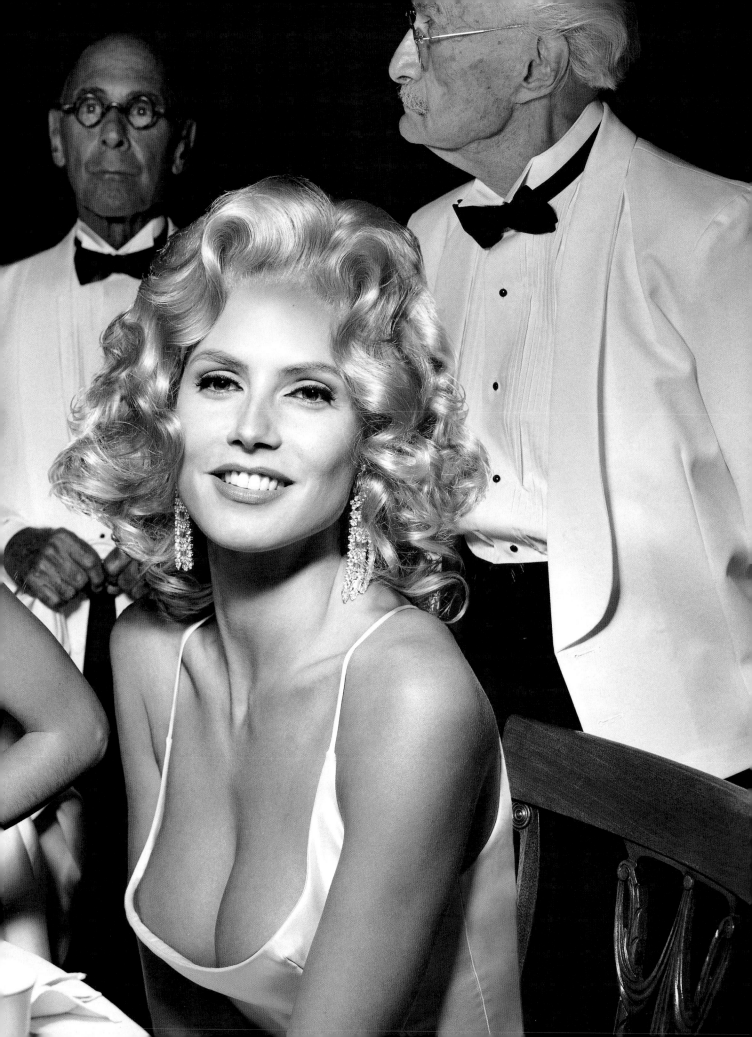

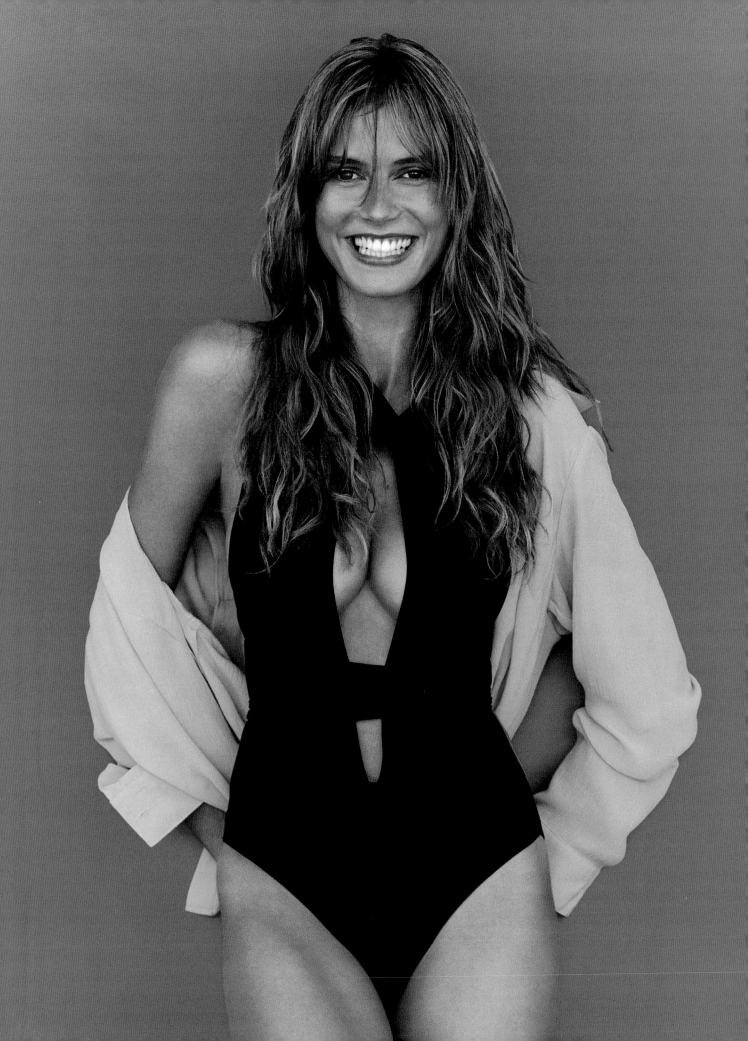

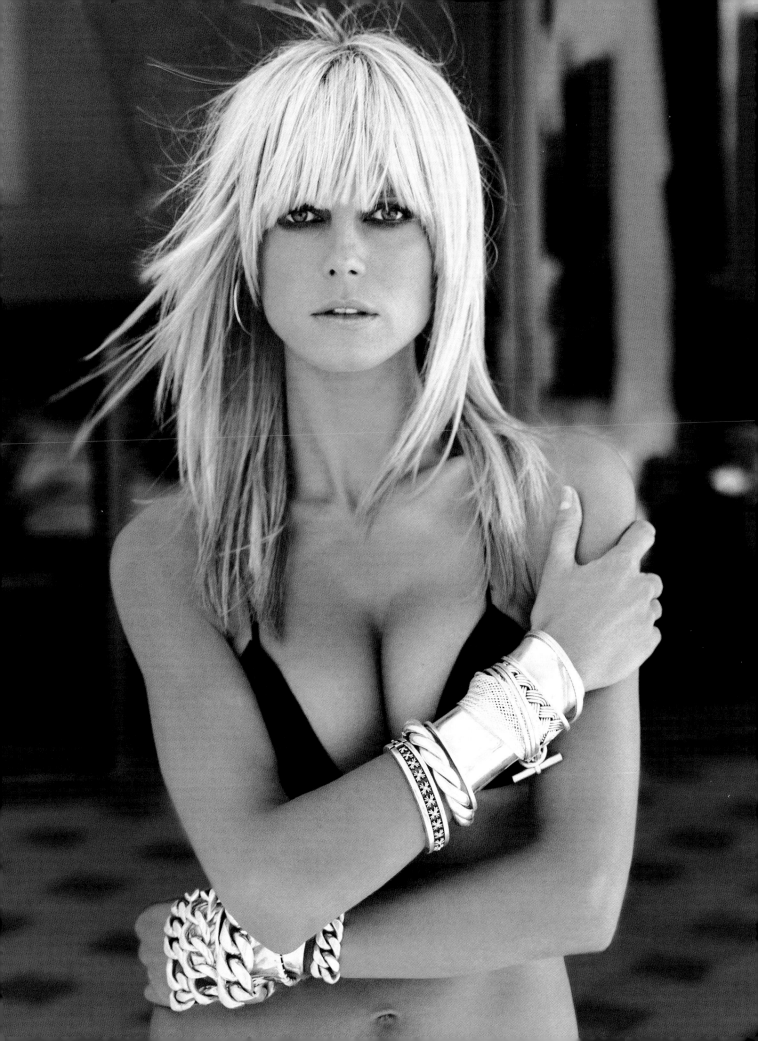

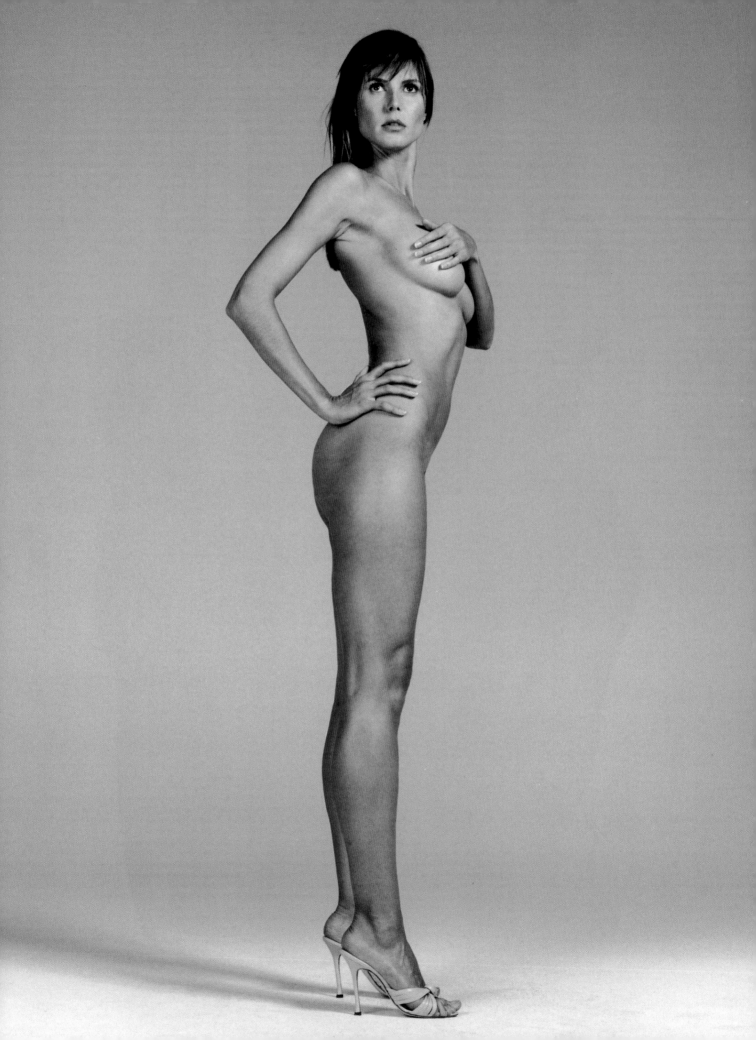

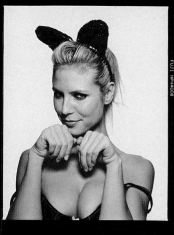
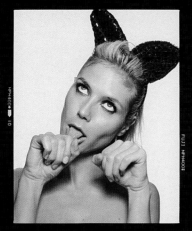
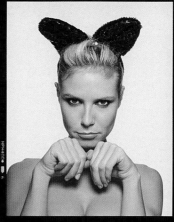
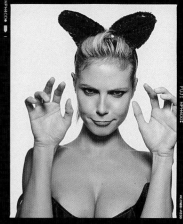
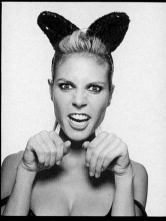
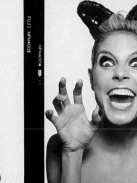
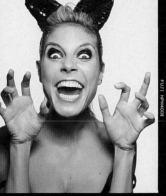
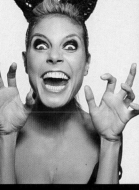
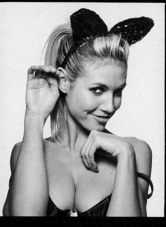
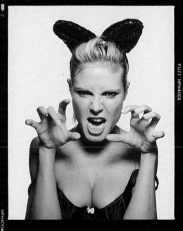
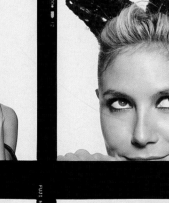
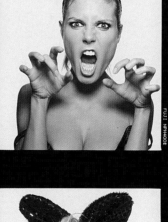
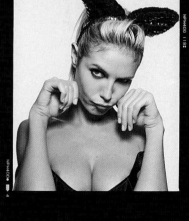
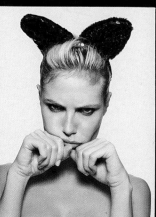
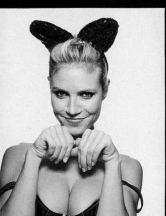
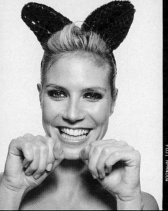
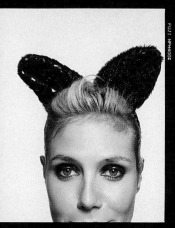

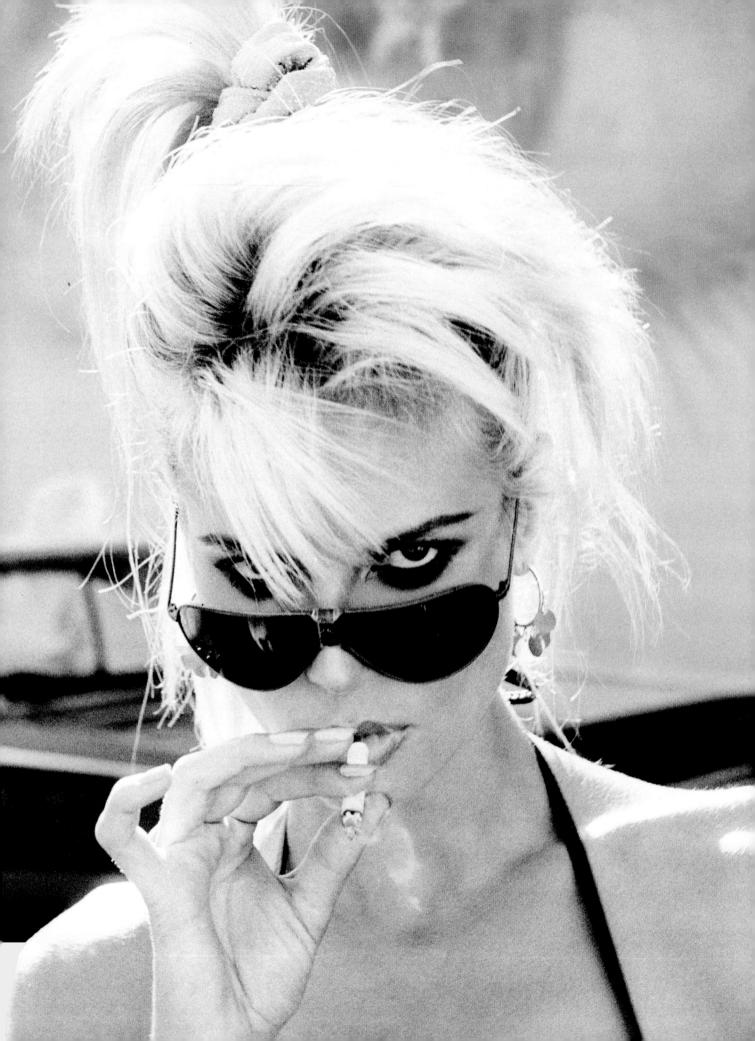

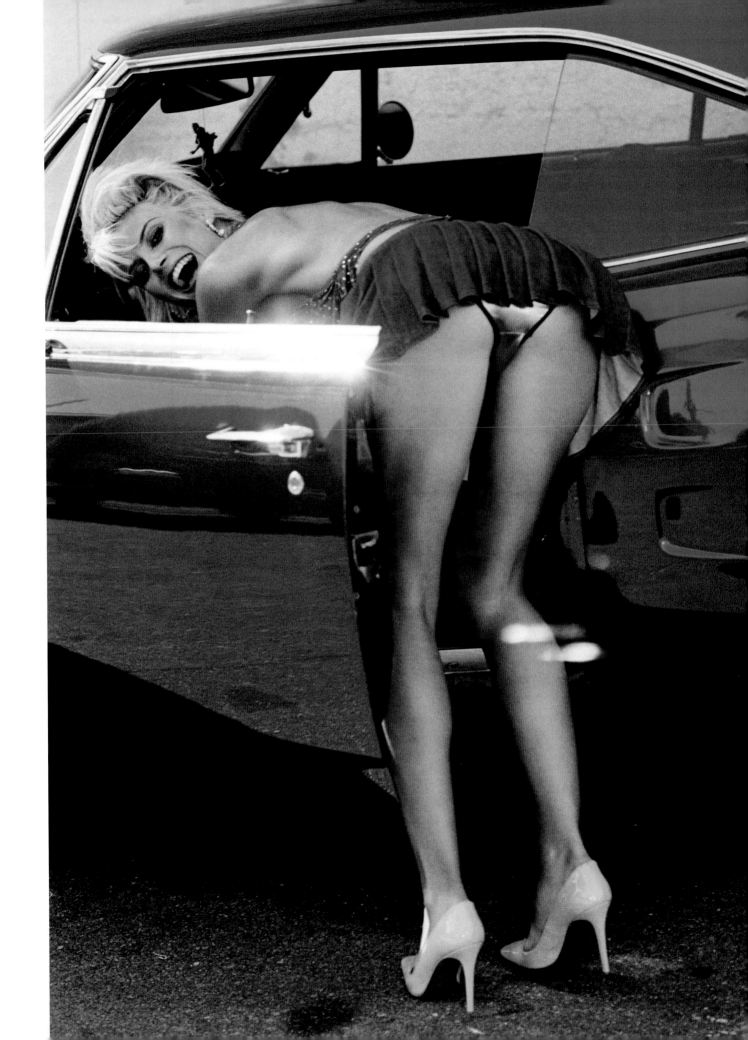

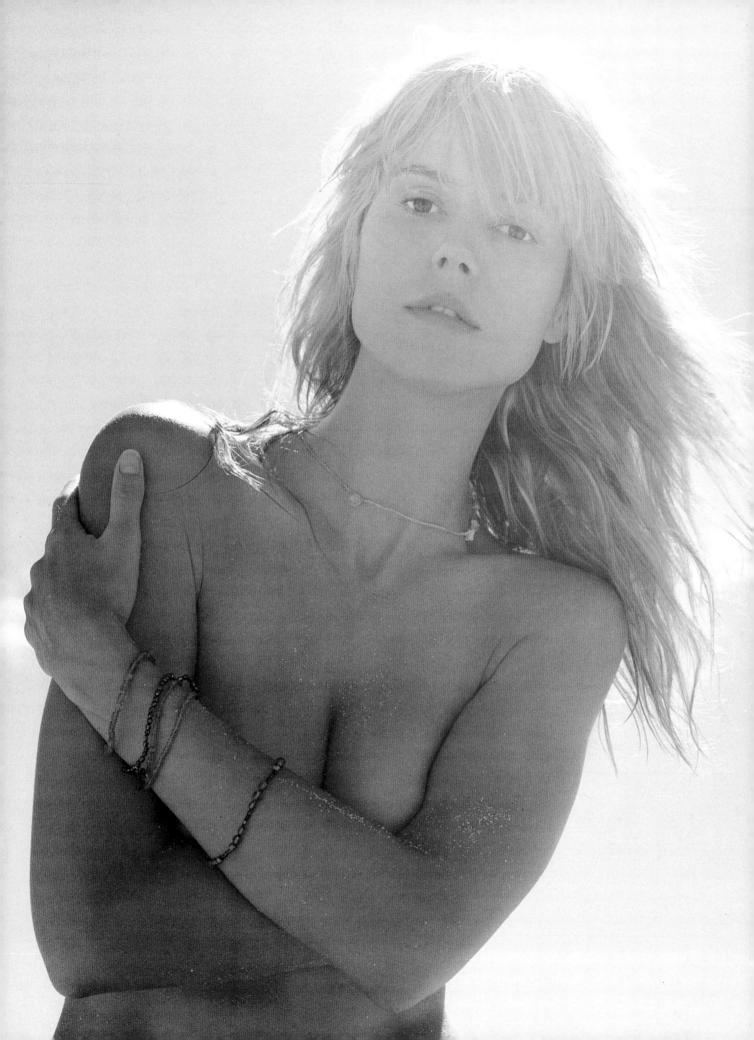

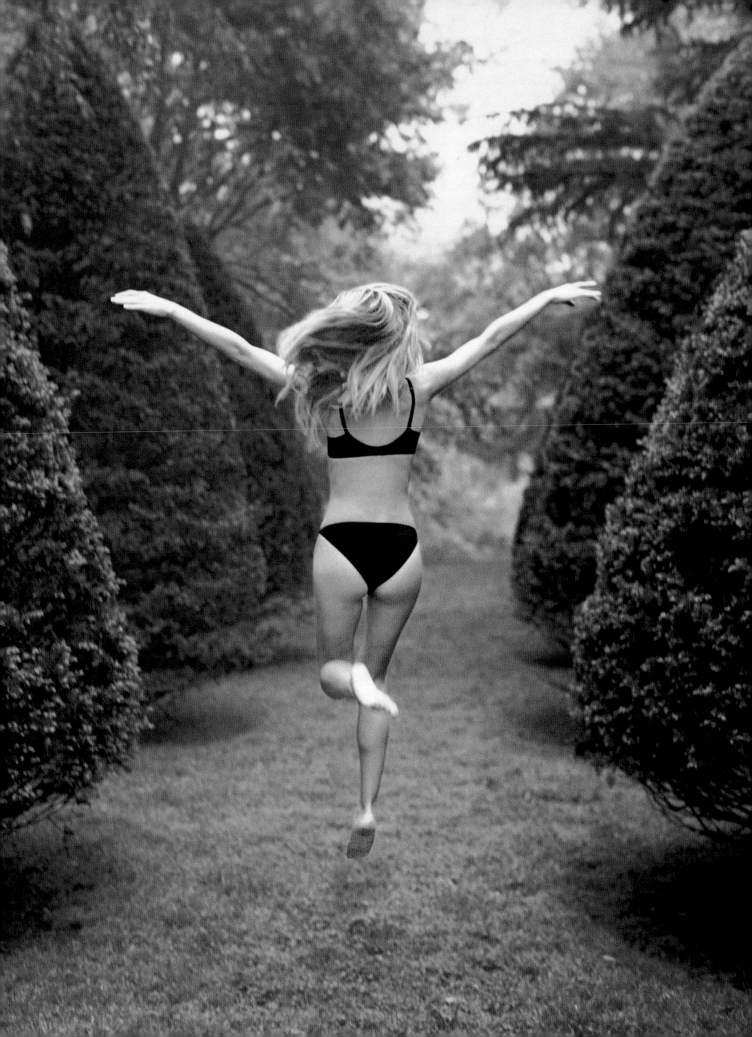

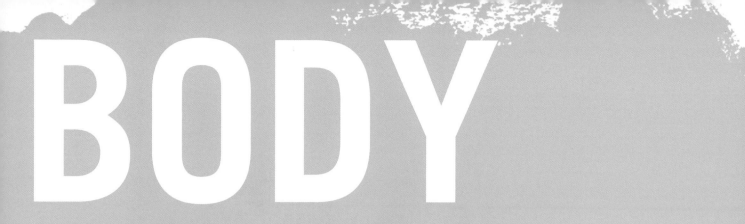

# BODY

**RULE 5**

shape it, be it

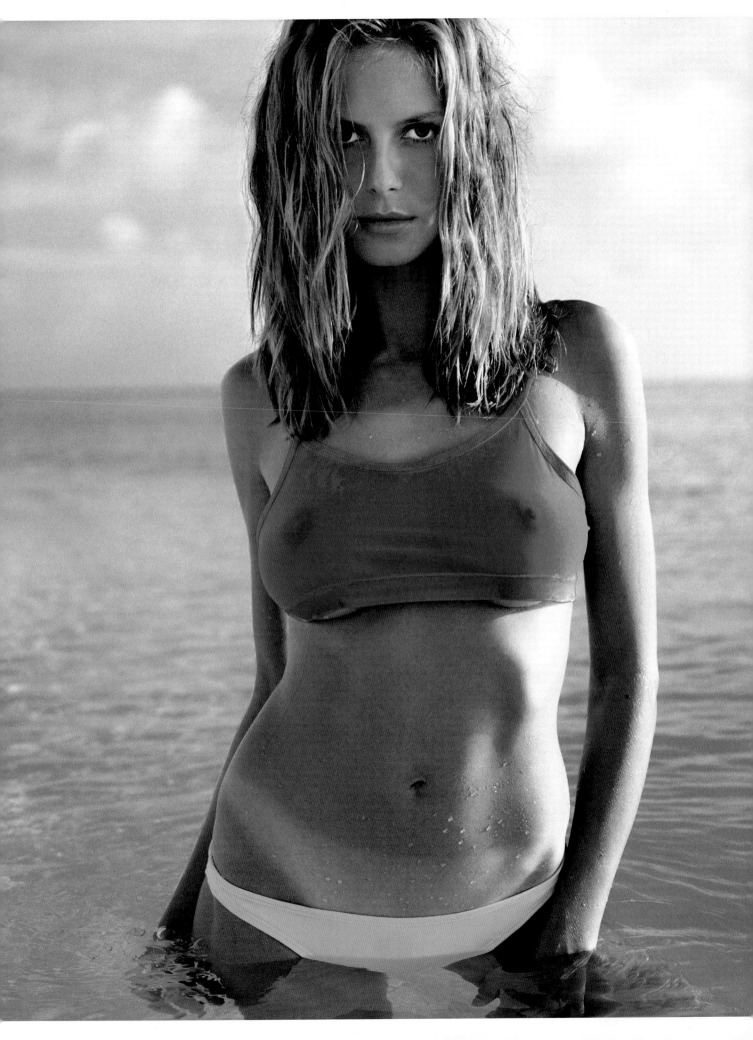

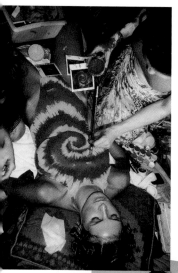

If someone had to be "The Body," I'm glad it was me.

Top models often become renowned for specific features—Christie Brinkley for her all-American smile, Christy Turlington for her dramatic bone structure, Linda Evangelista for her ever-changing haircut, Naomi Campbell for her fierce runway walk. For years, Elle MacPherson was known as "The Body": She's tall, athletic, and perfectly proportioned. Not surprisingly, she landed the *Sports Illustrated* swimsuit cover in 1986—and for three years after that.

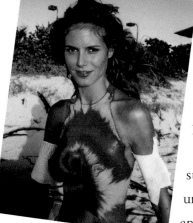

After the *New York Post* anointed me the new "Body" underneath my picture in their Page Six column (thanks again to Desiree), the impact was immediate: That day, backstage at the Victoria's Secret fashion show, lots of TV interviewers suddenly wanted to talk to me. Thankfully, I not only made it through my first runway show without falling or otherwise embarrassing myself, but "The Body" nickname stuck for a while. Later that year, I got my own coveted cover of the *Sports Illustrated* swimsuit issue.

The image I had of my body growing up was very different from the superconfident image I'm supposed to project now. It's not that I was uncomfortable with bodies—mine or anyone else's. Being raised in Germany and having traveled with my family around Europe where nudity on beaches is common, I'd seen up close the range of human bodies, tight to saggy, big to small.

Despite the endless hours—up to 12 per day—of body painting for *Sports Illustrated*, this was one of my favorite shoots.

As a girl I had wide hips, and I was flat as a board. At thirteen, my boobs began to appear . . . correction: My *boob* began to appear, since one grew first and faster than the other. Fortunately, the slowpoke followed soon after.

At the start of my modeling career, I tried hard to get work in Paris and Milan but, ironically, for a former string bean, now I just wasn't skinny enough. I'd walk into an audition all cheery —"Hi!"—and I could see the way they'd already scrutinized my figure (to me: healthy; to them: oversize) and written me off. There were models who took appetite suppressants, even drugs, to stay thin (though I imagine that wasn't the only reason they indulged). Models, like certain athletes, often do things to their body that "help" in the short term but may cause long-term damage.

Eventually, after I moved to America, I started landing better jobs. One of my earliest covers was *Self,* whose emphasis on healthy body types and self-acceptance

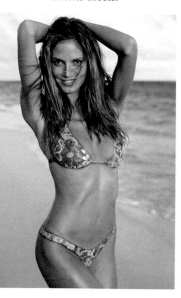

made me feel like their poster girl. I also appeared on the covers of *Fitness* and *New Woman,* two other magazines that weren't afraid to show a woman with healthy curves.

Clearly, there was a place for us nonwaifs in the business. I was thankful for that, since I'm proud of the body I have, and not embarrassed to show it.

Would I take off *all* my clothes for the camera? Actually, I have, for several photographs, but none where you could really see the Full Monty. When I posed for a somewhat risqué *Esquire* cover, a black-and-white nude plus a two-page, centerfold style insert by Matt Jones, my mother was a bit distressed. "Did you really *have* to do that?" she pleaded. But I thought it was a beautiful, sophisticated picture. Had there been even the suggestion of nipples or pubic hair, I might have vetoed it. Especially when it comes to nudity, it's important for me to have some control over how I am portrayed. There have been so many times I've 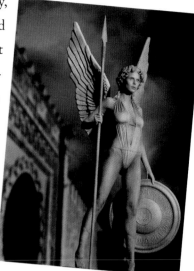 arrived for a shoot, especially for a men's magazine, and halfway through they've said, "Um, would you mind if, for this shot, you go topless and kind of clasp your hands over your chest?" I'm not naive, I know sex sells. But of course I *mind,* if it's something I didn't agree to from the beginning. You have to be strong and protect yourself. (I don't like being a jerk, but I've even had to ask fashion stylists who have called in only the skimpiest of clothes for a shoot to please find me something more modest.) Besides, if you're naked (or almost naked) in every picture, where's the mystery? People are going to get bored.

Another favorite picture of me in my birthday suit ran in the 1999 *Sports Illustrated* swimsuit issue, in which makeup genius Joanne Gair painted bathing suits onto us models. (Joanne was the artist behind the famous Demi Moore *Vanity Fair* cover in which a pregnant, naked Demi was painted from head to toe.) It took ten and a half hours of sitting, lying down, and standing (and trying to resist the urge to scratch) for Joanne to paint every inch of my torso so that I looked as if I was wearing a swimsuit. But I loved the results so much we went on to do two other body-painting shoots together.

Over the years, *Playboy* has called me a few times to pose. I've gotten all sorts of feedback from advisers and friends, ranging from "You absolutely MUST NOT EVER do *Playboy*! . . . Are you out of your ever-loving mind? . . . Don't you want to keep your dignity?" to "DO IT!! . . . Are you crazy? . . . You gotta do it!" My own reaction falls somewhere between those extremes. On one hand, *Playboy* is an American institution, and as a model I can almost see it as part of my career "checklist." On the other hand, it'd have to be done in a very particular way, one in which I'd have lots of control and could be proud of both the process and the final result.

I don't think there's anything morally wrong with posing nude. Some of the most beautiful pictures I've ever seen are nudes, even aside from the classic masterpieces. And I don't think there's anything shameful or harmful about nudity in and of itself. In fact, many years from now, I might like to have images of me in my entirety, during my "good old days," with my body in its prime, before gravity does the inevitable!

# beyond genes

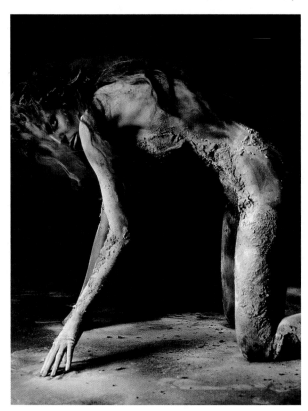

Obviously, looks are a model's stock-in-trade. Accountants had better be good with numbers; models had better be beautiful, youthful, and fit. And since everyone wants to feel beautiful, youthful, and fit, they see us as, well, the models of their physical fantasies. Because of that, lots of people assume that for models to look *that* thin, they certainly can't live normally and certainly, *certainly* can't eat normally. I promise you that not all models eat only rice cakes and salad leaves, or drink coffee by the pot, or smoke cigarettes by the carton. I have a huge appetite and a weakness for lots of "bad" things: bread, potatoes (I am German, after all), pasta (especially with cream sauce), candy (licorice chews, gummy bears, and chocolate with hazelnuts), hazelnut ice cream, full-fat yogurt with hazelnuts (are you detecting a trend?).

Oh, yeah. And I'm not particularly good about exercising.

But before this devolves into a finger-wagging lesson on how to exercise better, or a primer on how to eat better, or all those things that everyone's always carping at you to do if you want a better body, remember

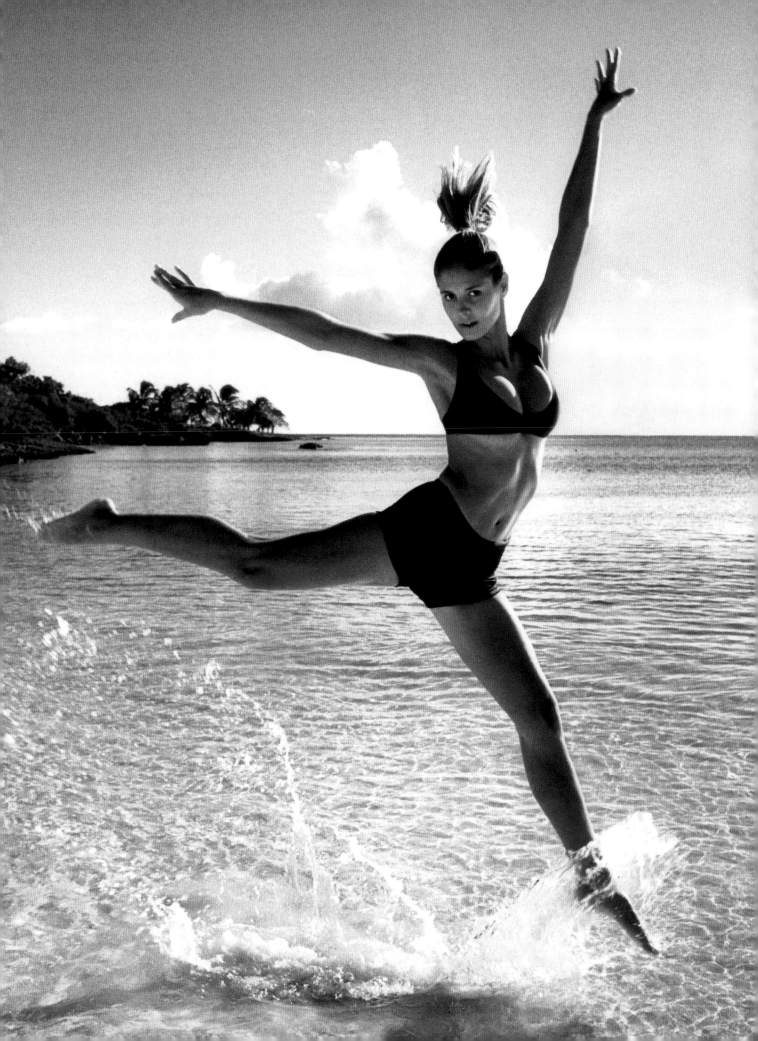

what is maybe the single most important rule of physical attraction: It's not so much what your body looks like, objectively. (Okay, so maybe it has *something* to do with that.) It has just as much to do with the mind: how you carry yourself; the vibe you give off; your swagger and carriage. Take my girlfriend Nina: She admits she isn't the skinniest person, but she has a nice body, wears sexy outfits, laughs all the time, enjoys life, dances like crazy. *That's* appealing . . . not locking yourself into extreme diets and crazy exercise regimes to the point where you no longer let yourself enjoy life's pleasures.

I hate when my trainer David Kirsch forgets his dumbbells at home and I have to carry him on my back. Don't try this at home!

## not my favorite subject, but let's do it: exercise

As I said, I'm not the world's most enthusiastic exerciser, but I've learned a few things over the years:

- *The older you get, the more you need to work out.* You know it, I know it—we get less limber, we injure more easily, we heal more slowly. All the more reason to try to maintain some level of fitness.

- *Workouts have to be fun* . . . or you won't exercise. If you don't like the gym, then run. If you don't want to run, then box. If you don't like to box, then have lots of sex. Whatever you're doing to burn calories, flex muscles, and boost your heart rate, make sure you enjoy it.

- *Exercise needs to be balanced.* Although at times it may be smart to pick a concrete "problem area" and make improving it your goal, you shouldn't work it to the exclusion of nonproblem areas.

Neglected muscles have a tendency to get together, say nasty things about you, and vow to rebel the first time you lean in for a pose you didn't do quite enough stretching for.

Just as it is with clothes, it's true with workouts: No one size fits all. Not everyone can get a rock-hard body or make any and all body parts look just the way we want. I, for instance, have a mushy German butt, and always will. First and foremost, I believe it's important to live a healthy life. Once you do that, you can get a lot closer to your ideal look. Sure, some of the enviable bodies out there have good genes going for them, but in most cases, those people also put more care into their bodies.

# THE "NO-SERIOUSLY-I-ONLY-HAVE-THIRTY-MINUTES" WORKOUT

BY DAVID KIRSCH, AUTHOR OF *SOUND MIND, SOUND BODY*

*David is a drill sergeant with heart. These exercises can work for anybody—anywhere.*

➤ **2 MINUTES:** Light stretching with knee bends

➤ **1 MINUTE:** Jumping jacks

➤ **30 SECONDS:** Platypus walk (Squat in wide stance with hands behind head, knees aligned with toes, butt sticking back. Walk forward while pushing off with each heel. Looks silly but it's a killer.)

➤ **1 MINUTE:** Shadowboxing with crossovers, uppercuts, knee bends

➤ **1 MINUTE:** Plié squats with calf raises (Squat with toes turned out at 45 degrees. Stick butt back as you squat down, keeping body weight in heels. As you sink into squat, bring heels off ground, rise onto balls of feet. Bring heels back to floor and shift body weight back into them, squeezing inner thighs and glutes before pressing back up.)

➤ **2 MINUTES:** Lunges

➤ **1 MINUTE:** Squat thrusts

➤ **1 MINUTE:** Scissors reverse crunch (Lie on back, bring legs into air to form 90-degree angle with body. Keep abs tight, bring feet apart to form scissor shape, pull from hips into a crunch.)

➤ **2 MINUTES:** Donkey Deluxes (On all fours, inhale and lift right knee toward chest. Exhale and press right foot back and up behind you in arcing motion. Inhale and lower leg until thigh is parallel to floor. Exhale as you raise leg again, to a 90-degree angle, pushing heel toward ceiling. Inhale as you lower. Now the left . . .)

➤ **1 MINUTE:** Sit-ups

➤ **1 MINUTE:** Push-ups

➤ **REST FOR 1 MINUTE** (no more, because you want to make this as cardio-intensive as possible; it's a circuit, after all): Drink water, repeat. If you're ambitious, do the sequence three to six times. If you have ankle weights or dumbbells, use; if not, no problem.

Okay, I'll grant you, if you really, *really* hate exercising (or you're really, *really* busy, or you really, *really* have three little kids to take care of), then even thirty minutes is tough to come by. If you're *that* time-strapped, try:

➤ **DOING SIT-UPS** right after getting out of bed, before starting the day

➤ **KICKING YOUR LEG OUT BEHIND YOU AND SIDEWAYS** while brushing your teeth (it works the hamstrings and butt)

➤ **TAKING STAIRS INSTEAD OF ELEVATORS,** and always taking them two steps at a time.

It's insanely easy to fit *some* kind of physical activity in—and you don't even have to get near a piece of Lycra.

Women, especially, get huge pleasure from having a great physique: It frees us to wear more body-conscious outfits, it makes men look at us more, and because we feel sexier, it makes us feel more powerful. I don't know how much extra willpower the typical model has, but because it's our job to be in great shape, and it's the way we make money, we have built-in motivation that others don't. My point?

> The biggest obstacle to getting a really good body is your own brain.

I won't give you one of those obnoxious exercise regimens to follow. I'll just tell you how I work a little fitness into daily life. I sweat it without sweating too much, if that makes sense.

Because I travel so much, it's hard for me to get to a gym on a regular basis. So I'll call David Kirsch, my trainer, and he'll fax me a routine when I'm in Europe, for example, that I can do even in my hotel room or outside before a photo shoot. David is the author of the book *Sound Mind, Sound Body.* He runs the Madison Square Club in Manhattan, and he has lots of good ideas about health and fitness. He's been able to convince me (and others) that if we don't want to work out for too long, it's important to make every second of the routine count, and the way to do that is to "engage your mind." By zeroing in on the body part you're working, you get more out of the exercise.

## it's not just about salad

Along with working out, of course, it's important to eat well—or at least better than you probably do. Often I feel that, if I haven't worked out one day (or the next, or the next), so long as I've eaten smart, exercise isn't imperative. (Note to cardiologists and fitness gurus: Please don't write to berate me. I'm just being realistic.) Yeah, I've tried various diets—carried my juicer all over the world, ate cabbage soup every day for a month. But better than dieting is just developing healthier eating habits.

In one long exhalation, here's everything I try and do to eat well: I stick to fruits, vegetables (the darker the green, like kale and spinach, the better), salads, chicken, fish, yogurt, eggs. I've stopped eating most red meat. As for volume, when it's healthy stuff, you can eat lots of it. I stay away from chips and peanut butter and bread, especially white bread that has pretty much zero nutritional value. I think before I eat that candy bar I don't totally need. I try not to eat on the run. I should drink more water than I do, and David is always barking at me, "Are you hydrating?" I take vitamins. I absolutely stay away from fat-free stuff. I try to avoid fried food. I steer clear of too many additives.

Perhaps watching and helping my mother and grandmother cook when I was a young girl—cutting off the ends of beans, washing and chopping vegetables, whipping up sauces, learning how to make sauerkraut soup (see page 135 for the recipe)—all of that made me at least aware of what goes into the body. If you think of what food does to you and for you, you naturally want to eat better.

On the other hand, though my mother and grandmother cooked, I can't say that every dish was healthy. So many of the meals were heavy—potatoes, meat, cream sauces. A perfect example: my grandma's *knödel*. She'd shred raw potatoes, put them in a pillowcase, put the pillowcase in the clothes dryer to spin out all the moisture, add salt and egg, and boil it, which produced this potato mush, which she then formed into potato balls . . . but wait! She then made a sauce by cutting bacon into tiny bits, frying them, then drizzling the potato balls with the fat and

I love room service. You know that saying, "Her eyes are bigger than her stomach?" Somehow I always seem to manage.

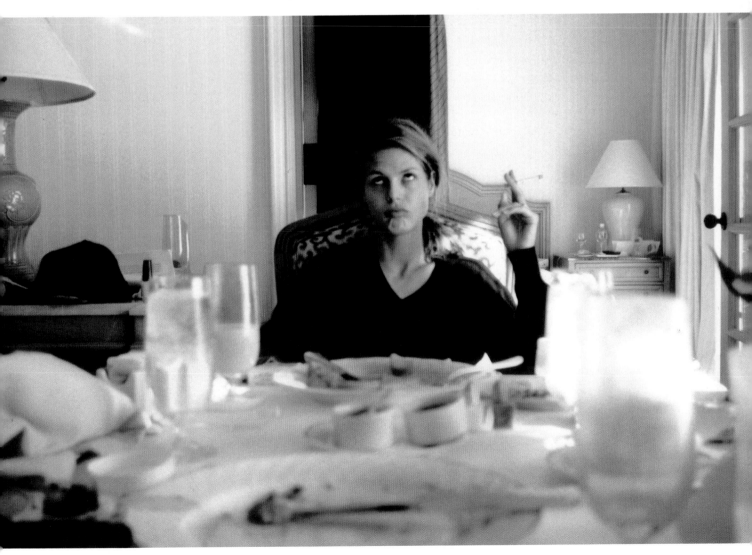

bacon bits. Yummy? Unbelievably. But probably not something they'll be serving on spa menus anytime soon.

# pleasure on a plate

So many girls I see, in and out of the business, are underweight. Recently, at a runway show, I hugged a fellow model and couldn't believe it. There was no meat on her! When I squeezed, I literally heard the sound of bones crunching.

I chose to be the way I am instead of starving myself. At the Victoria's Secret shoots, there's always a gigantic smorgasbord—pasta, trays of desserts, chips, huge bowls of candy, assorted types of jerky—and I can see that many of the younger girls, who are less sure of themselves, are afraid to eat in public. Me, I don't really care about that, or what they say about me. In fact, I've been known to order a pizza backstage. On the other hand, if I have a runway show coming up and I've gained a few pounds, I can get it off in two weeks so long as I go cold turkey on the "bad" stuff—bread, rice, potatoes, sugar, Coke, and especially those daily Starbucks lattes foaming over with milk.

Almost as important as what you eat is *how* you eat.

## SNACKS YOU CAN PACK

*When you grab food on the go, better to eat something that works for your brain as well as your metabolism—and fills you up so you don't get the munchies again right away.*

**1.** Instead of chips/pretzels/candy, snack on raw almonds. They have a ridiculously high density of vitamin E (higher even than avocados) and fiber. And they contain polyunsaturated fat—the *good* kind of fat.

**2.** Pop blueberries. They have the highest concentration of antioxidants of any fruit; they're low in calories, high in good flavor.

**3.** If you're flying, bring trail mix or carrot sticks to kill your appetite, because plane food is not designed for the health- and diet-conscious (unless you're flying Air Weight Watchers).

**4.** Most of us don't like drinking water, so flavor it—with lemons, oranges, cucumbers. Or drink herbal waters and teas. Green tea, particularly decaffeinated, and mint tea are just as hydrating as the stuff out of the tap.

**5.** Protein shakes—100 percent whey protein, made with water instead of milk—are nutritious and filling. They contain a mere 80 to 100 calories, they're fat-free and carb-free, and full of protein. Throw in a handful of berries for flavor.

## MY GRANDMOTHER'S SAUERKRAUT SOUP

A great dish for a party; serves 12 as a main course

1½ lbs. ground beef
1½ lbs. ground pork
5 large white onions, chopped fine
2 tablespoons olive oil
3 cans (14–16 ounces each) sauerkraut
2 cans (6–8 ounces each) sliced mushrooms
5 whole sweet pickles, chopped rough
1 12-oz. bottle Heinz Chili Sauce (or regular ketchup)
2 quarts broth made from 4 vegetable bouillon cubes
Salt and pepper to taste
1 small (8 oz.) container heavy cream

1. Sauté ground beef and pork and onions with olive oil in a soup pot until brown.
2. Add sauerkraut and mushrooms (with their liquids) and pickles; stir together with the meat.
3. Add entire bottle of sauce or ketchup and the vegetable broth.
4. Simmer for 45 minutes, stirring occasionally.
5. Add salt and pepper to taste.
6. Add heavy cream and cook for 1 more minute, then serve.

A woman who just moves her fork around the plate is not fun; a man with such a woman is probably not enjoying her company; a man who eats less than you is just plain weird. When you're dining with people, or on a date, or at a party, or any kind of celebration, show that you can take pleasure in food and eating, because that shows how you can take pleasure in other things.

Oh, yeah: And when you're *not* eating, don't talk about what you've been eating. Nothing's more boring than that.

Even though my image has appeared in many fashion magazines, I encourage you not to let what you see in those pages determine what you should wear or how you should look. Decide what's right for *your* body. The more comfortable you are with yourself, the more attractive you'll be—to men, to women, and to yourself.

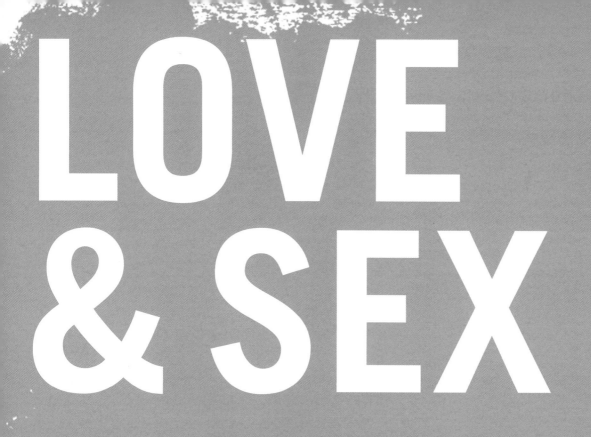

# LOVE
# & SEX

**RULE 6**

*become*

the fantasy

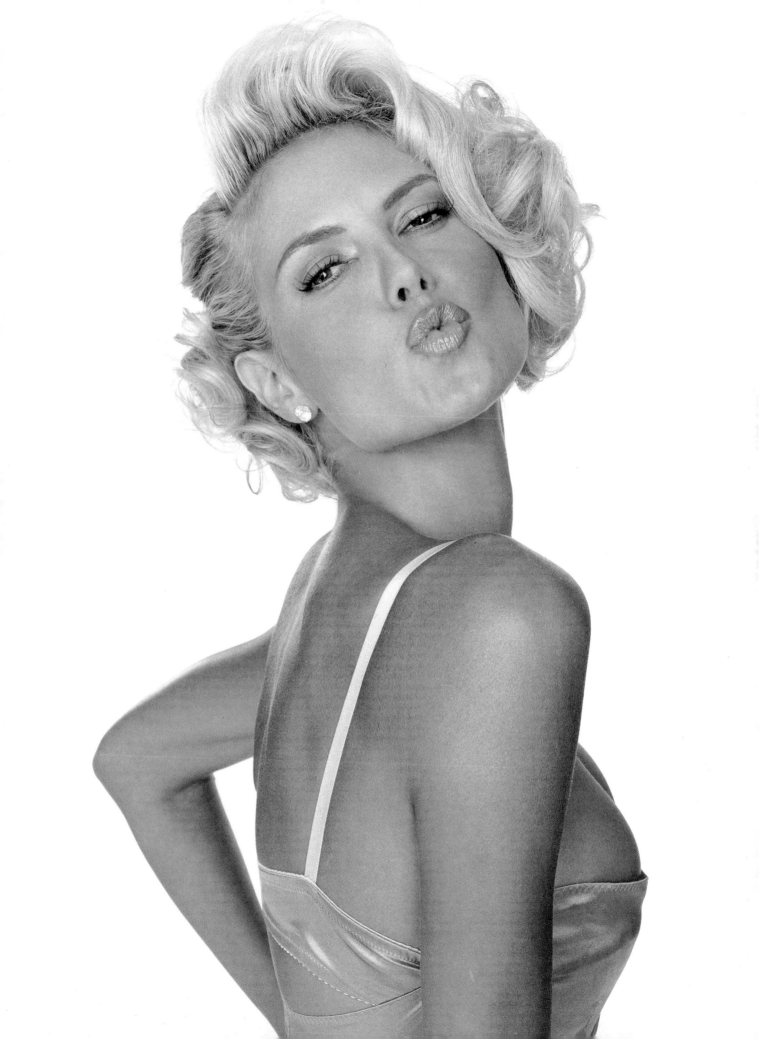

**P**rofessionally, it's my job (among other things) to simulate stimulation, fanning the fantasy that anything is possible: that I can be yours, that you can be me—heck, that *I* can be me.

Romance? An endless series of candlelight winings and dinings.

Sex? It must be blow-the-roof-off hot.

Love? Well, love . . .

Love's a different matter. Love is the real thing. We all want love, and models are no more or less successful at it than anyone else.

I don't claim to be a love expert. In relationships, I've been the dumper and the dumpee. I've had good sex and great sex. (You know that quip about how sex is like pizza? When it's great, it's great, and when it's bad . . . well, it's still pretty great.) But I've been lucky enough in my life to have loved truly and been truly loved.

For five years, I was married to a wonderful man, celebrity hairstylist Ric Pipino. We had so many amazing experiences, living and growing as a couple. Of course we had the typical arguments of couples: With a model and a hairstylist, you can imagine that getting ready to go out to a big event was always good for some back-and-forth bickering and last-minute style changes. But there was undeniably a certain comfort and security in being married—in feeling that someone's got your back, you've got theirs, and you're unified in having to make decisions ranging from who drives or which dry cleaner does the shirts better to big-picture stuff like whether to have children, or sadly, whether to stay together.

I learned a lot from Ric. And actually, as with any strong or intense relationship, we ended up learning a lot together—about compromise, patience, understanding, and not sweating the small stuff. I'm not saying that we learned those lessons perfectly or always gracefully,

Ric and I were together for seven years. During that time, we grew a lot and shared many amazing experiences. . . . That time of my life will always be special.

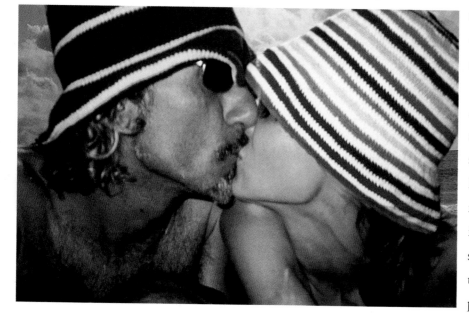

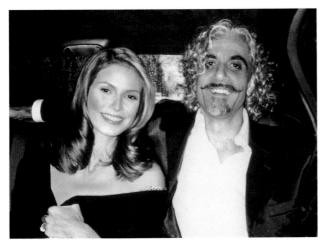

but I can honestly say I grew in the relationship. Life sometimes leads two people, even ones who are close, to different points where it becomes clear that it's best to part ways, but I'll always be thankful that I had someone like him in my life. I actually don't know that I'll ever get married again . . . but we'll see. I know that I'll always be an optimist, a romantic, and a lover of love.

So I know love's the real thing, and not a subject for flip commentary. There are also many steps leading up to it that demand thought and feeling and even work. But they also hinge on having enough confidence in your fantasies to make them realities.

# why her? why him?

The mind is an erogenous zone. To prove it, just look at models: Why do some people respond to one model more than another? Is it just aesthetic preference (this one has bigger boobs, that one's a redhead)? Of course not. Sure, that plays a part, but who we desire is much more a reflection of the wanter than it is of the wanted.

My first boyfriend, an achingly cool fourteen-year-old who drove a moped, won my twelve-year-old heart one sweltering summer afternoon when we spoke through a chain-link fence at the local swimming hall. We would ride all over town—to the movies, park, festivals—and make out for hours on end. (This was in the early days of hysteria over AIDS contagion, and after each kissing session we'd go to a public bathroom and wash out our mouths so we wouldn't catch the disease!) With his wheels, his muscular adolescent build, and the masterful way he had of extinguishing his cigarette, he embodied the freedom of adulthood that seemed to be just around the corner, and I was totally, completely in love.

Then again, I'm always head-over-heels for the one I'm with. I love being in love—that butterfly feeling in your gut, not wanting to do anything else but be with that person. If I don't at least believe I'm in love, I find it difficult to open up to someone, to have sex, to want to pursue the next step. If my first boyfriend was true love, so was the second, and the third. Each relationship was completely different, and each one in its way contributed to who I am today. At one point, I dated a guy who lived in the Italian Tyrol, near where my family rented a ski house. I truly believed that he and I were going to get married, live in the mountains, open an inn, and have a flock of children. I looked forward to my life as a Tyrolean house-

## OBJECTS OF DESIRE

| THE MALE FANTASY | THE FEMALE FANTASY |
|---|---|
| Championships | Relationships |
| Manual labor | Manolo Blahnik |
| Ordering for both of you | Eating for two |
| Making deals | Finding sales |
| Rock-hard abs | Rock-hard abs |
| Sports by satellite | Bath by candlelight |
| National security | Personal freedom |
| Holding off on the climax | Luxuriating in the climax |
| Always knowing what to do | Always knowing what to say |
| Improved job title (and respect) | Respect (and improved job title) |
| Not crying | Not regretting |
| Channel-surfing | Chanel-surfing |

wife, making beds and cooking up meals for the crowds of skiiers who'd come through—until finally *he* convinced me that I'd never be happy. The first guy I dated when I came to America was (I thought) true love, even though I didn't understand a word he was saying.

> Every relationship teaches you something unexpected.

It teaches you something about yourself, about how love works, about what you will and won't settle for.

I'm not necessarily recommending therapy to figure out what's behind your romantic choices. *(Why do all the women I'm interested in look like my mother? Why must I be with a guy at least ten years older than I am?)* If the man who rocks your world is a banker and social wallflower, then that says something about you, and that's cool. Is your dream mate someone who, first and foremost, you need to have fun with? Someone who'll take care of you? Someone you can mold? The potential for romance isn't killed by understanding what you need in a partner and why. In fact, if you understand your choices better, maybe you can manipulate your circumstances so that you have a better chance of meeting someone. (For example, if a guy who doesn't make a lot of money is a nonstarter for you, no matter how drop-dead gorgeous/brilliant/funny/warm he may be, then perhaps you should stop bar-hopping Friday and Saturday nights with your poet/dancer/origami-teacher friends.)

# cruise control

There's nothing harder than putting yourself out there, no matter what you look like, or what the odds are of success. If you don't have the nerve or confidence to go out on that limb, let me direct you back to Rule 2 (Sell It!) to remind you how, in order to take more control of your life, you need to *act* nervy, *act* confident. I know a woman who, whenever she sees a guy she likes from afar, says to herself, *He's going to be with someone. Why shouldn't that someone be me?* Now, that doesn't mean she always approaches the man, or that if she does, she goes to bed with him. It means she's got an attitude that gives her confidence to feel she has as much right as any woman to talk to him and make him aware that she exists.

Nothing's going on in your love life? Why not? Examine that. Have you been hiding at home watching videos? Always hanging with the same crowd? Has your sex drive gone into hibernation?

You have no excuse for not putting yourself out there. Simple as that. If you see someone you're interested in and do absolutely nothing about it, you might never see that person again. That might have been your match, or at least a very good match, and you'll have missed the train.

For a woman to make the first move is admittedly tough. It's not the norm, and it can be uncomfortable to court pure, unadulterated rejection. (I give you males of the species big-time props for what it must feel like to always put yourselves out there.) But that doesn't mean you shouldn't try. You empower yourself by creating opportunity. And hey: A lot of men out there love that take-charge attitude. (And lots of other men can't handle it.)

Note to men: When trying out an opening line, really think about what you're going to say before anything comes out of your mouth. Ask yourself: Where could this get me? Where do I *want* this to get me? What possible answers could she give? For instance, a compliment is always nice. But asking about astrological signs is gigantically lazy, and the "Have we met before?" approach is just dumb. I'm not saying that to deliver a pickup line you should play a whole chess game in your head, thinking five steps ahead. But would it be so hard to think, um, one answer ahead? My point—for your benefit as much as hers—is: Don't ask a question that could easily lead to a dead end. Yes, you never know where a conversation's going to go, but a little anticipation wouldn't kill you. If nothing else, it tells her that you're not the sort of guy who, thirty seconds after first meeting, wants *her* to take charge of the conversation (and everything else, should the meeting heat up and lead someplace).

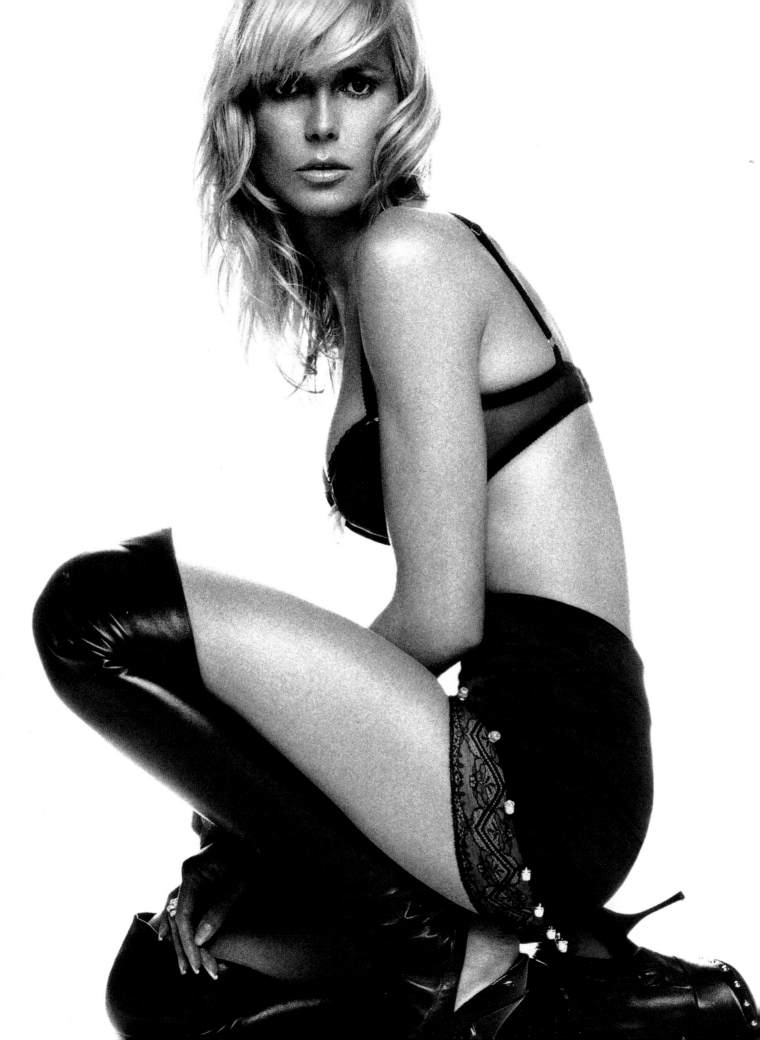

## A FEW THINGS MEN MAY NOT KNOW ABOUT WOMEN'S DESIRE

**1.** No matter how much she protests, she wants to be taken care of.

**2.** She doesn't dress sexy just for you.

**3.** She wants you to feel slightly threatened by her success.

**4.** She loves diamonds. Even tomboys love diamonds.

**5.** Sometimes, a woman wants to be told what to do . . . especially in bed.

**6.** She really does think that women would do a better job of running the world.

**7.** When she's fantasizing, you're right: It's not generally about hot sex. But don't think hot sex doesn't play a part. Or that you're always the protagonist, you silly little man.

**8.** She's got sides to her that even she hasn't yet seen (no, that doesn't mean she's got multiple-personality disorder).

**9.** If it were a choice between her having a great body or her man having a great body, she'd take the great body.

## A FEW THINGS WOMEN MAY NOT KNOW ABOUT MEN'S DESIRE*

**1.** No matter how much he protests, he wants to take care of you.

**2.** Even if he fantasizes about other women, he wants you to fantasize about him.

**3.** If you're not fantasizing about only him, then at least fantasize about some perfect abstraction of a guy who does not and cannot possibly exist . . . then apply all of your incredible desire for Mr. Nonexistent Perfect Guy to him.

**4.** He really believes The Perfect Girl for Him (aka The One) is out there.

**5.** He's often distant because no one ever told him exactly what it would feel like when The One appeared in his life, so he's not always sure if you're It.

**6.** He needs to believe that *you* believe he's capable of great things (whether he is or not).

**7.** He wants to be reassured without asking for it.

**8.** If you reassure him too much without his asking for it, he worries.

**9.** If it were a choice between having a great body or having a woman with a great body, he'd take the babe.

(*or so I hear)

There are other common pickup scenarios doomed to fail, many of which we women still scratch our heads over. In an effort to rid the world of these world-class losers (the approaches, that is), I thought I'd point them out so that maybe you'll think twice (or a thousand times) before using them again.

• Whistling after us, like we're dogs. What do you expect us to do—bark?

• Using suggestive wordplay/double entendre about our anatomy or a sex act ("Can I see your tan lines?" "Are you a real redhead?" "Cold out, isn't it?"). When you do this, a neon sign appears right above your head that flashes LOSER . . . LOSER . . . LOSER . . .

• Inappropriate excess. Recently, I met a guy for all of two minutes in Los Angeles. He sent me diamond earrings with a note: "Bling-bling . . . I think you look really hot . . . I wouldn't mind hanging out with you." Sweet. Oh, yeah: And he was married.

That's a lot of man bashing—so let me now say something nice about guys. There's one particular character trait that many of you possess (though some of you don't always use it) that's extremely redeeming: good old-fashioned respect. I'm not saying a man has to joust with another man to prove his love for a woman, or throw his expensive jacket over a muddy puddle so she can cross without ruining her Jimmy Choos. But while I don't want to rely on a man, or be just eye candy on his arm, I do believe I should be treated well. Especially if I've just met a guy, he should hold the door for me, and let me go through first. Outdated or not, it's a kind of respect

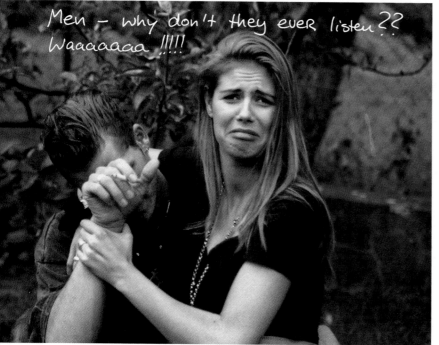

and treatment that women (for the most part) want and respond to.

On a date, for instance, don't talk about yourself so much (a particular peeve of mine). Ask about *us*—where we're from, our family, our interests, our life goals. Not only does it make you seem like a gentleman, and someone interested in things other than yourself, but it gives you information you need to know anyway, right? You'll quickly learn whether we're the girl you want to live your life with, the girl you just want to go to bed with, or the girl you can't ditch fast enough after the check comes.

# supreme courting

Of all the early aspects of a growing relationship—flirting, meeting, getting to know each other, romancing—it's the last one that best represents what we models do: sustain the dream. That's really what romance and courtship are about, no? Romance promises to keep the flame going, makes things fun, mysterious, alluring, seductive.

Romance is so simple—and not necessarily what you think. It just requires a little imagination and empathy. It's not about flowers and chocolate and jewelry and tickets to a great show and swell dinners (though, for the record, our feelings about those are, in order, nice, nice, nice, nice, and nice). In lieu of all those long-stemmed roses—and for a lot less money—why not:

- *Make something?* Anything. A homemade thingy or even a heartfelt card (with a poem written by you, not Hallmark) will be treasured.
- *Lie in bed and talk?* Give cuddling a chance. Really.
- *Cook her dinner at home?* Plan, shop, prepare, set the table, serve, enjoy with her, clean up afterward. (Write only to tell me you *didn't* get lucky.)
- *Give her a whole day to herself?* Insist she indulge in all the solitary and/or girl things she loves to do and rarely has time for. She'll come home refreshed, grateful, probably horny.
- *Go dancing with her?* And if you know or can learn a few traditional steps (not just the white-man's-overbite-disco thing), you'll be amazed how erotic it can be. (Write only to tell me you *didn't* get lucky afterward.)
- *Make plans, any plans?* That is, take the initiative to schedule an event (getting tickets to see a limited-engagement show at the museum, or planning a B&B weekend away or a hike, etc). Too many guys just come home, plop on the couch, turn on the TV, and say, "Hey, babe—so what are we doing this weekend?"

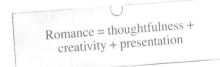

Romance = thoughtfulness + creativity + presentation

Maybe the best thing about romance is that it's a pleasure in itself. Just by doing it, you get happy, while also paving the way for bigger and better things. If you follow some of the suggestions above (or, way better, come up with your own homemade ideas), I feel that most of you, in the near future, will be getting very lucky.

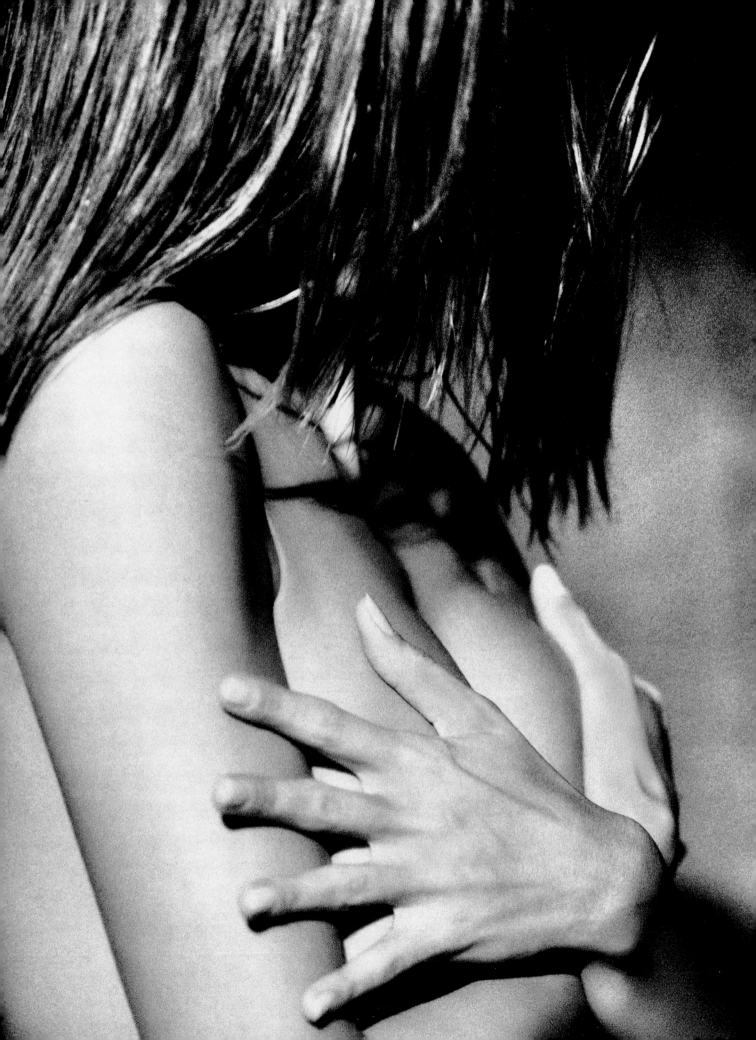

## SO YOU REALLY WANT TO MEET A MODEL?

**1.** Be six foot three and look amazing naked.

**2.** Go where models congregate—New York, L.A., Miami, Paris, London, Milan, St. Barth's—and hit the hottest restaurants and clubs (if they're listed in the guidebook as hot, they're not). Even better, wrangle an invitation to a restaurant or club opening. Some PR agencies hire models to show up as desirable "guests."

**3.** Don't introduce yourself with "You must hear this all the time, but . . . " If I hear it all the time, what makes your version interesting?

**4.** Act confident but not lascivious. In fact, act normal. We're accustomed to meeting too many narcissistic guys who think we'll like them because they look good in Calvin Klein underwear.

**5.** If I smell your cologne before I see you, you're wearing too much.

**6.** Spending more time talking on the cell phone (even if it's "to Europe") than to the person you're with is not cool.

**7.** Don't touch—not even a hand, shoulder, or knee—unless you're very, *very* sure it'll be well received (i.e., after you've gotten back lots of smiles and eye contact or some touching from us first).

**8.** Don't hide a wedding ring in your pocket. Really. Don't.

**9.** Don't take walks with someone else's dog or someone else's kid if you're, say, allergic (to dogs or to kids). I mean, a charade can go on only so long, right?*

*True, pretty much all this advice (with the exception maybe of #2) can easily be applied to your meeting anyone, not just models. Let's just consider it a public service announcement to help anyone who hits on women (and the women who are hit on). As for the meeting models thing? It'll never happen.

## let's talk about sex

I won't get into nuts and bolts and arms and legs and tongues here. But relationships get more exciting—for your partner and for you—when people talk about their fantasies, or ask what their partner's fantasies are.

Lots of women hedge their bets, and don't express such naughtiness; many women *never* say what turns them on. Good soldiers that they are, women will do all these things that their men desire them to do, but do we just want to have sex so that *he* has pleasure? Sounds unfair to me. So then how do you get yourself in the mood for love, or in the mind frame to try something new?

The same way I get in the mood when I'm on a bathing-suit shoot, my knees planted in the sand and cold waves slapping my back. Or when I've squeezed into

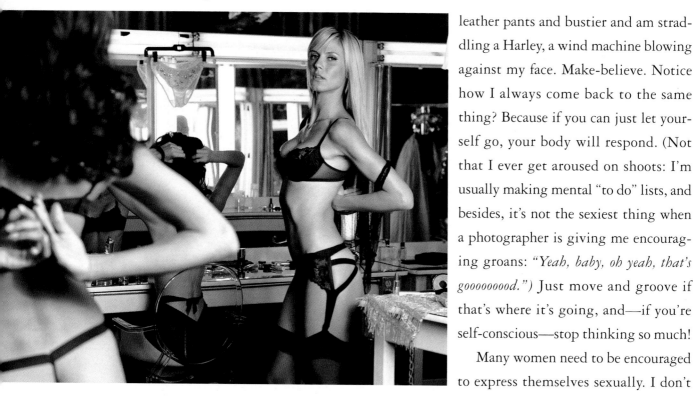

leather pants and bustier and am straddling a Harley, a wind machine blowing against my face. Make-believe. Notice how I always come back to the same thing? Because if you can just let yourself go, your body will respond. (Not that I ever get aroused on shoots: I'm usually making mental "to do" lists, and besides, it's not the sexiest thing when a photographer is giving me encouraging groans: *"Yeah, baby, oh yeah, that's goooooooood."*) Just move and groove if that's where it's going, and—if you're self-conscious—stop thinking so much!

Many women need to be encouraged to express themselves sexually. I don't mean you suddenly become this horny creature specializing in pole-dancing (though he'd probably enjoy that), but you want to do things *together,* grow with him, become a different, more fulfilled person. Maybe this comparison isn't completely relevant, but whenever I'm preparing for a TV appearance or a movie casting, I'm terrified, and wish I didn't have to go. Afterward, of course, I always feel so glad that I did. Point: If you always do the same thing, you won't grow. You wear different outfits every day, so why not try different sexual techniques?

Surprise is an aphrodisiac.

Since you only live once, get as much pleasure out of sex as possible, and get it on your terms.

How about naughty lingerie or garter belts—ever wear them? If not, why not? Do you have sex only in the dark? If so, why are you inhibited with the lights on? Have you ever been tempted to act out a favorite seduction scene from a movie or book? No? How about the same scene using a hilarious foreign accent? Does he come, and then you come (or maybe not) . . . and then you both immediately go to sleep? When you think of doing something outrageous that you've never done, why haven't you done it? Embarrassment for yourself? For your partner? Embarrassment that you might like it? How often does the fantasy recur?

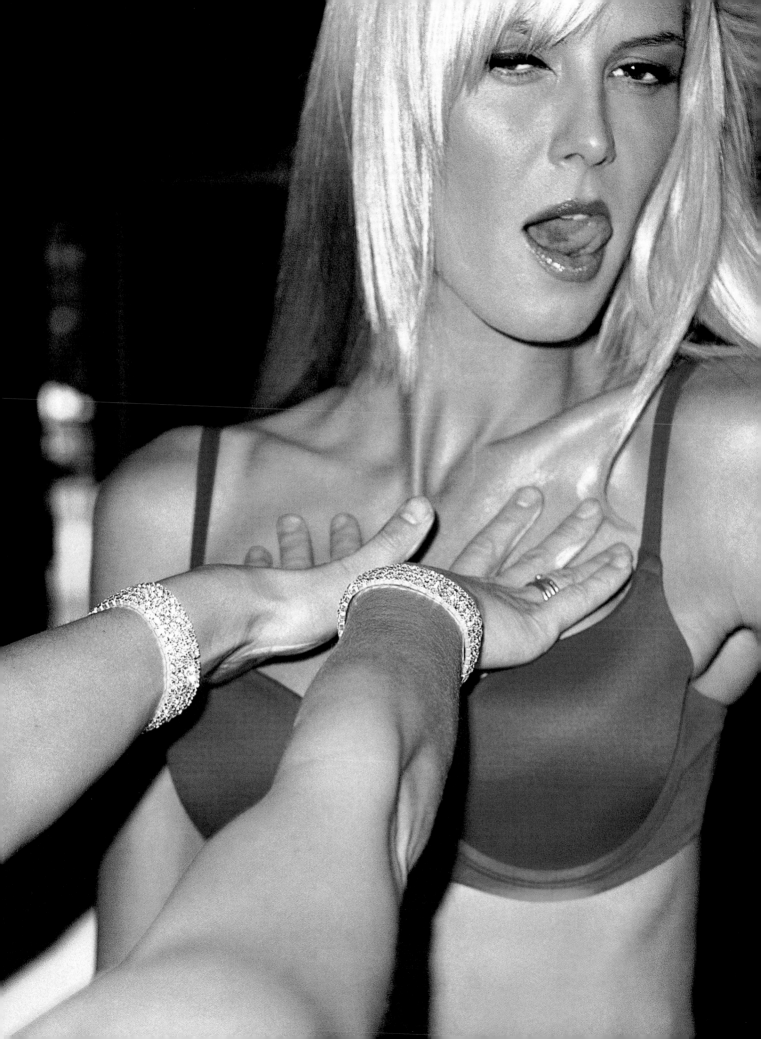

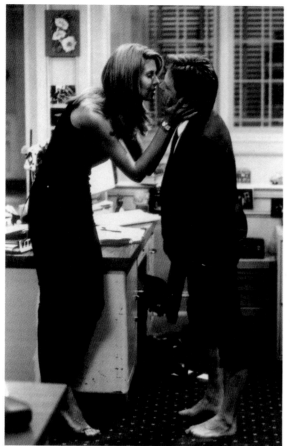

## MY FIRST KISS

Okay, so I mean my first *on-screen* kiss.

I found myself on the TV sitcom *Spin City,* where I played Michael J. Fox's love interest for six episodes.

I quickly fell in love with Michael. He's the sweetest man on the planet, this dream guy I've loved since I was little and first saw him in *Back to the Future.* Now, here I was years later, on the set of a prime-time American TV show, and suddenly I had to do all these intimate things with him. Because he's so good at what he does, and so comfortable doing it, he just chatted away easily about his personal life, while I was deeply focused on my lines. I marveled at how he could just talk about normal things and then, all of a sudden, when they yelled "Action!", he could do exactly what he was supposed to do, perfectly.

When it was time for our kiss, I asked if we were supposed to actually kiss in rehearsal. We were. (There are worse things . . . ) To sell it, I had to make it look like I was really into him (which, given my affection for him, wasn't hard), but I was also scared about kissing someone I didn't know. And, of course, there were cameras everywhere.

To meet his mouth, I had to bend down: Not only am I quite a bit taller (he's five feet four, I'm five feet nine), but I was also wearing heels, so the difference between us was even greater.

I bent down until I was level with his cute little face. He did not have a big mouth. But still, there was that "kissing problem": You can't go straight at someone. I started turning red. It seemed to go okay.

We had to kiss several times. We ate a lot of mints. He would pop in a mint; I would pop in a mint.

Later, there was a scene where we're in bed together, post-sex. Just when the scene started, I started to . . . yodel. (The producers knew I had this talent and had suggested that if I unleashed it at just the right moment, it might get a good reaction.) "What are you doing?" Michael asked.

"I always yodel after sex," I said.

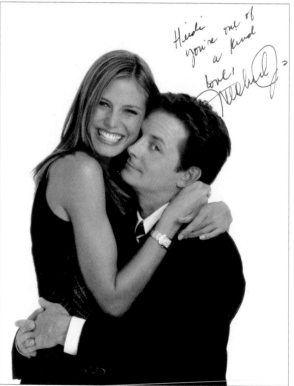

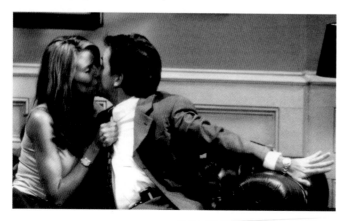

What I mean is that women, in particular, have to be honest with themselves and their partners about what they want, or else they're always going to be the ones serving up the show. It is, after all, called "making" love—there's an element of creativity to it. And even if you use the more antiseptic, male vocabulary, they're still known as sexual "acts." An act requires imagination, a performance.

# fan the flames

If you're lucky enough to have commitment and security as well as lots of freshness and excitement and earth-shifting sex, raise a glass of champagne to you and your partner.

But one of the biggest challenges to romantic love, certainly, is how to keep it exciting once the newness has worn off. Personally, I think living together is the most challenging aspect to marriage. When we get comfortable with someone, we tend to stop making an effort, and find ourselves going to bed each night in sweatpants and big old granny undies, with cold cream on our faces. Or bustling through the day expressing little more affection for each other than a rote peck on the lips. Just because you're in a happy rhythm doesn't mean that you no longer need explosions of joy and surprise.

If you still want the big payback, then you have to make the effort. My personal fave is to leave lipstick messages on the mirror, or secret love notes and Polaroids stuffed into pockets or suitcases. It also slays me when my man writes me a love poem—it doesn't have to be good, just from the heart. So maybe you don't do rose petals strewn on the bed; you can still light scented candles. Maybe a love poem is too ambitious; you can certainly whip off a midday e-mail that says "I'm thinking about you naked under your lingerie, except for the part about the lingerie." Maybe you don't have the money to go to some romantic bed-and-breakfast; you can still call your honey at work, insisting she or he meet you downstairs for an illicit frappuccino. Don't settle for plain vanilla sex: Do it in the shower, in the kitchen, just inside the front door when one of you gets home from work.

The more *new* things you do together, the more interesting your history together will be, and the more interesting you'll be to each other. By the way, that's one of the things I love most about vacationing with a sweetheart: Because you're not at home following your routine, you're sort of forced to do original, even risky things (if you've never tried skinny-dipping under a star-filled sky, you must). On the other hand, if you're on vacation and find yourself saying things like, "Ooh, let's not do that, I don't want to break my nails" or "I'd rather not get dirty" . . . you really need to take a vacation. From yourself.

I'm not suggesting you completely make over your personality for love. I *am* saying that you can improve on things to give yourself more of a chance to be happy in your romantic life. If you're shy, you may never get out there on the dance floor, or be a chatterbox at a party, or wear crotchless panties. If you're a tomboy, you're not going to turn yourself into a Playboy bunny. But being a tomboy doesn't mean that you never bring out your femininity. Being shy doesn't mean you always let yourself get passed over. You can change in a way that still feels appropriate and natural to who you are.

Everyone can make their lives better—their romantic lives, too. You just need to figure out what it is you want, come up with a reasonable plan, and follow it. There's no reason you can't live (and be) the fantasy.

## QUEER EYE FOR THE STRAIGHT GIRL'S SEX LIFE

*Look, we know that guys are much more eloquent talking about the shortcomings of their favorite football team's defensive ends than about what turns them on in bed. So I consulted a gay friend of mine, let's call him Mr. Big (no, not that one), to give us some tips on how to pleasure our men in the sack. Here are Mr. Big's top seven tips. Oh man. I'm going to live to regret this one:*

**1.** The first thing that's crucial is how you gauge your partner's response to your touch. For instance, if you try a light tickle, like you'd do behind a cat's ear, then you must read the person, by the expression on his face, and decide whether he likes it more delicately or more aggressively.

**2.** Make eye contact. Whether you're touching or changing positions, eye contact establishes greater intimacy.

**3.** Try synchronizing your breathing at times—heavy breathing's good.

**4.** Men are very sensitive on their nipples. But don't bite! Licking is good; blowing is nice. That drives men wild.

**5.** Never demean your partner's masculinity. Comparisons are not helpful. As far as you both are concerned, you're the only people in the world at that moment.

**6.** Massage is a good icebreaker. You have to be really delicate, like with the tip of the finger, and touch behind the knee, on the thigh, the nipple, the stomach. Every once in a while, you can get a little more overtly sexual, just to drive them a little crazy, and then you can stop again and just massage.

**7.** Sex is, of course, really visual, so try having a go in front of a mirror. And it's verbal, too. Be free to be vocal and don't worry about saying the "right thing." But the good thing about sex is that while you're performing it, everything is allowed. You needn't be prudish about it. If you want to have amazing sex, you should go for it. You have to be adventurous, within your comfort level. Every encounter can be a learning experience.

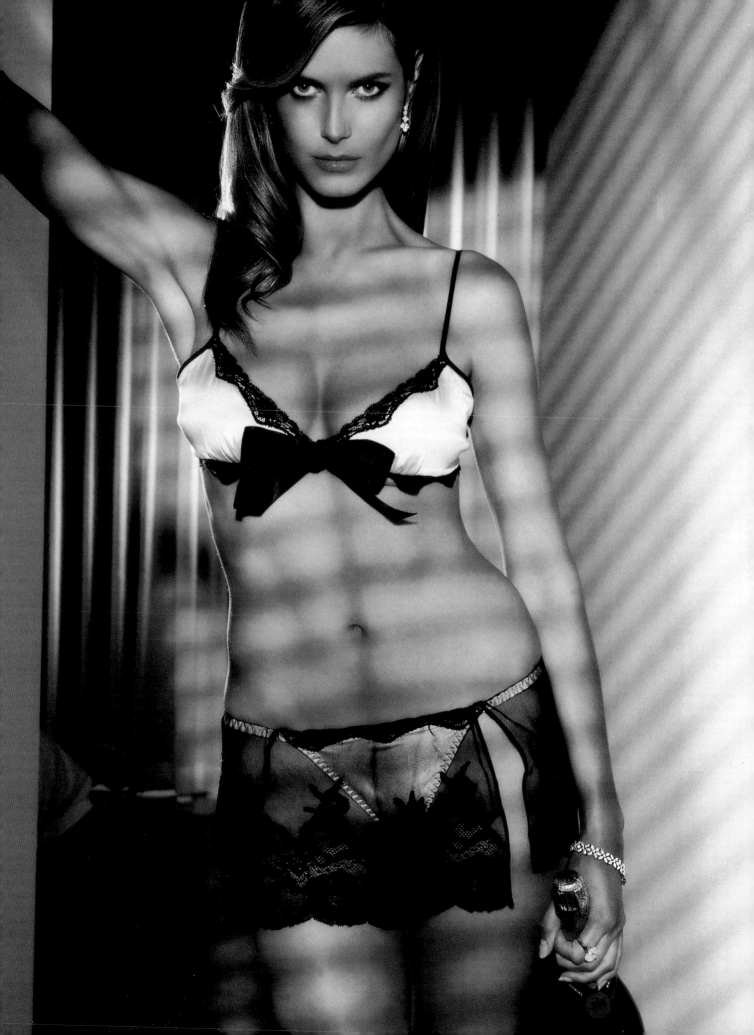

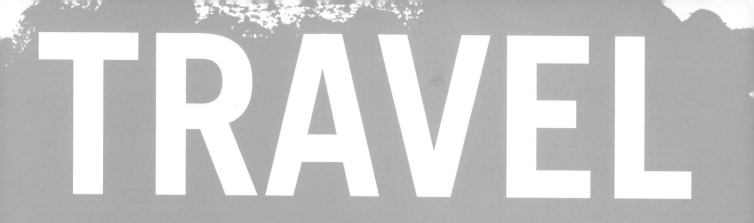

# TRAVEL

**RULE 7**

*be a* jet-setter

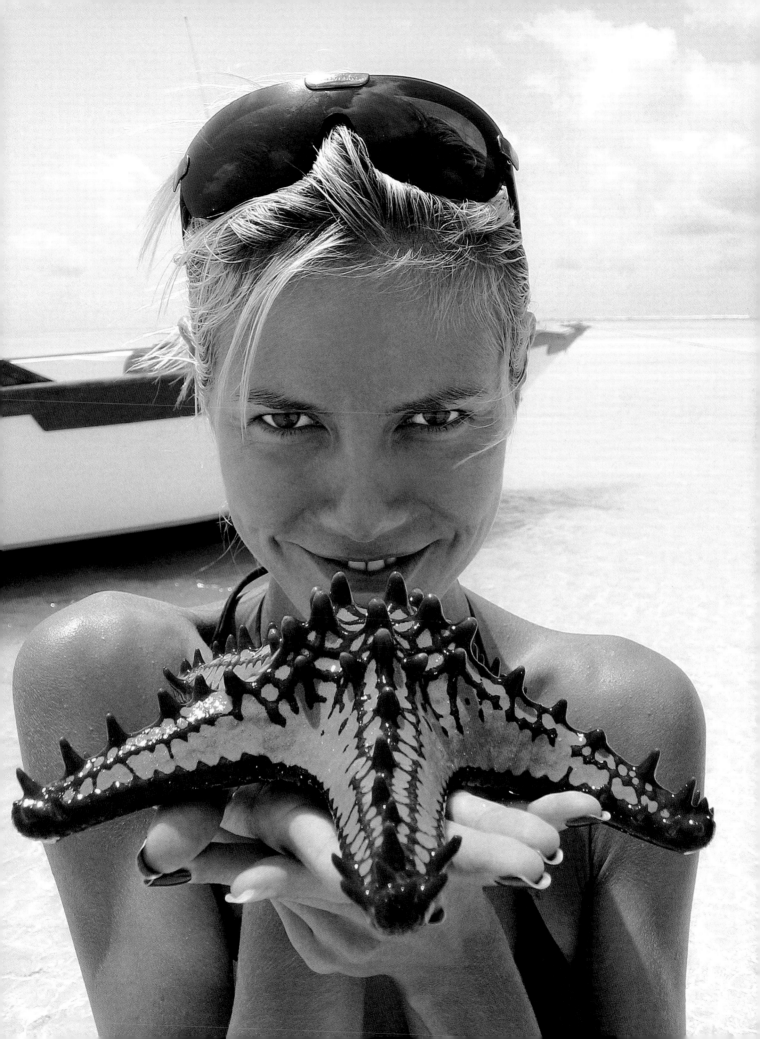

**S**o there I was, on a dive boat in the middle of the Caribbean, watching the dark shadows of fifty reef sharks moving through the murky water. My first-ever dive lesson had been all of twenty-four hours earlier, and now I was being outfitted with fifty pounds of scuba gear while being instructed to just "step off" the side of the boat. Right into where the teeming sharks were.

As the *Jaws* theme song repeated in my head, I wondered how I'd gotten myself into this.

When Discovery Channel had asked me, months before, if I would tape an episode of "Shark Week," I'd said sure—that abstract "Yeah, why not?" answer you give

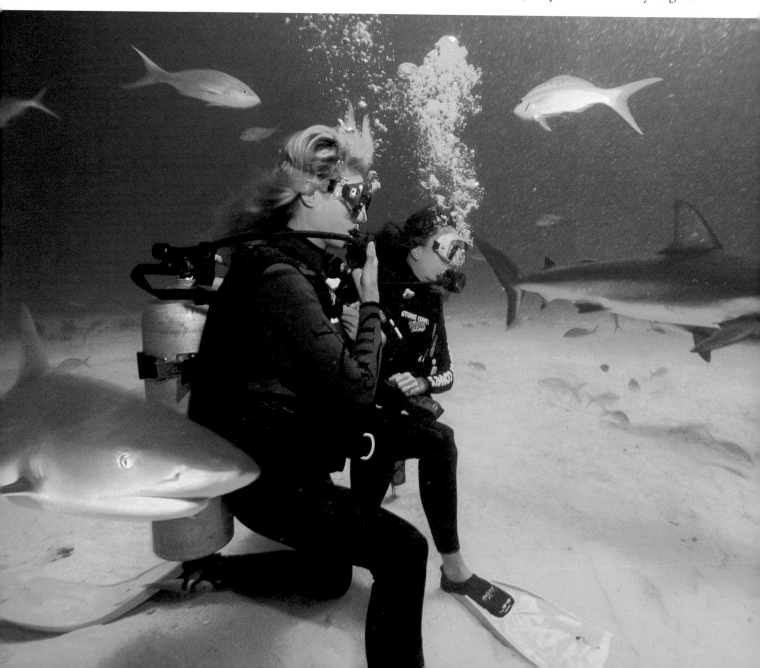

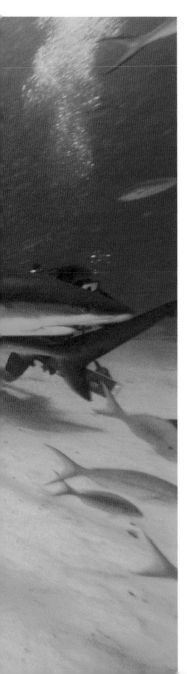

when you're being polite and noncommittal. A couple of weeks later, my assistant got a call asking for my exact measurements for a customized wet suit, and did I prefer window or aisle on the flight to the Bahamas?

In the weeks leading up to the trip, I told myself that this was another "fun" adventure I'd look back on with fondness and wonder—that is, after the absolute paralyzing fear had subsided.

But now, as I was being thrown to the sharks—literally—that self-pep talk seemed hollow, and doomsday scenarios fought with one another in my mind, like sharks going at chum. After all, everyone always tells you that *usually* nothing goes wrong. *One-in-a-million chance that something bad could happen . . . It's so unlikely, it's ridiculous even to think about it. . . .* My concern soon devolved into paranoia, and I was deep at work on my conspiracy theory—that the plan all along was to have the sharks come after me, so that they'd have "Supermodel Gets Mauled" on camera. Imagine the promos—the ratings would be spectacular, right?

While I indulged my paranoid delusions, all the dive instructors and producers milled around me saying, "It's happening . . . push comes to shove . . ." and suddenly I heard a countdown—*10 . . . 9 . . . 8 . . .* I had my goggles and fins on, my mouthpiece and regulator. I remembered how Nigel the Animal Wrestler, a lunatic who wrestles snakes and crocodiles for fun, told me that even *he* gets scared doing what I was about to do *. . . 7 . . . 6 . . .* Oh, and if you jump in and accidentally land on top of a shark? *. . . 5 . . . 4 . . .* They may feel threatened and bite you, so *do* be careful *. . . 3 . . . 2 . . . 1 . . .*

And so I went.

Was I surprised. Once I got down there, I was amazed at how beautiful and peaceful it was. The sharks, mostly larger than I am, were majestic creatures simply swimming by, not bothering with us humans so much as letting us know in their quietly commanding way that this was their turf. I imagine it's the closest I'll ever get to feeling like an astronaut in space, surrounded by stillness and orbiting shadows. It wasn't scary once I was safely planted on the ocean's sandy bottom, observing the sharks in their natural environment. Still, I was glad I wasn't the one hand-feeding them raw fish guts—especially when I heard, later that night, that on the dive right after ours a shark turned frisky, captured the feeding spear, and bit one of the feeder's arms (shrouded, fortunately, in a steel-mesh protective glove).

Now, from the perch of hindsight, I can say that swimming with sharks was an eye-opening experience, a beautiful memory. Which is exactly what travel and seeking adventure are about. As much as any aspect of my job as model, I'm most grateful for the chance to meet people in far-flung places and to experience other ways of

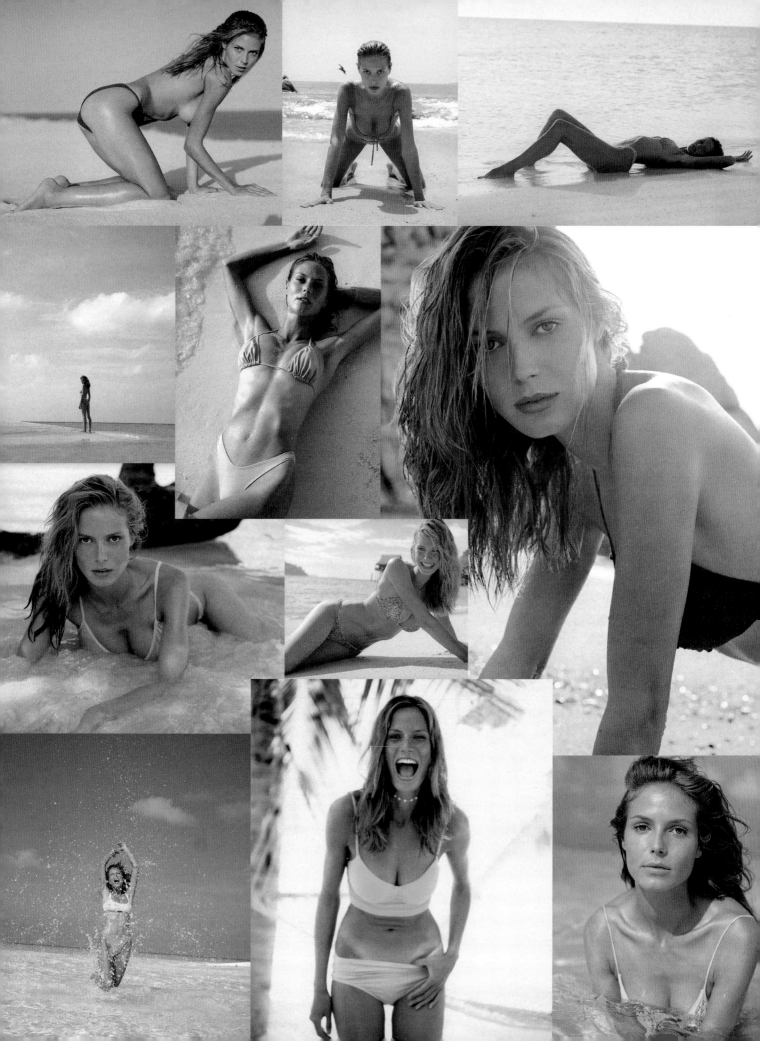

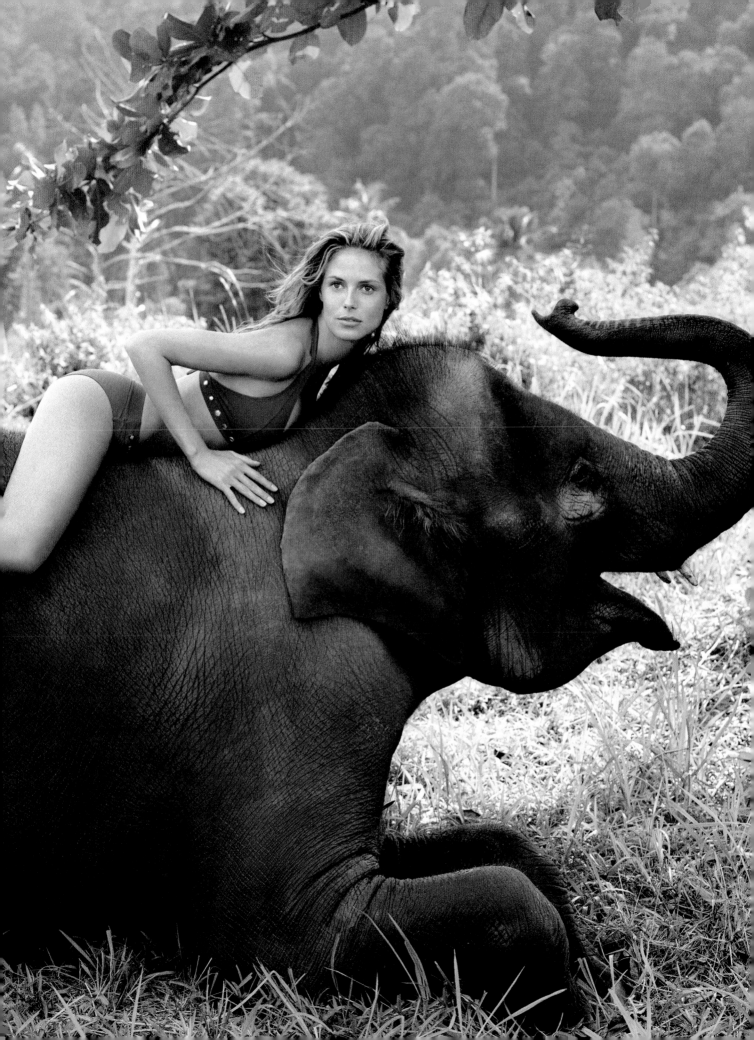

being. There's simply no travel book or TV show that can capture the true sense of what a place is like. Watching people in their homes, walking the streets, chatting with strangers, eating unfamiliar foods, just taking in the smells, sights, and sounds of a new place—all of this helps get you out of that rut.

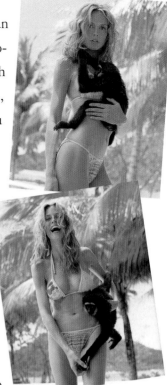

I've traveled the world and been asked to do some pretty wacko things for my job. On occasion, I've had doubts about being so adventurous—for instance, when on a single *Sports Illustrated* swimsuit issue shoot in Malaysia, I was quite literally thrown to the beasts. First, I rode an elephant with no saddle, wearing nothing more than a bikini (nobody told me that elephants are nearly as prickly as porcupines). The elephant got stung on his foot by a bee and bolted, with me holding onto his back for dear life. Later, I lay in some brackish water as a huge python constricted its full length around my torso (meantime, the monkeys in the trees above us were screaming, flashing their teeth, and generally freak-

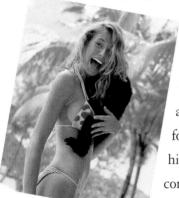

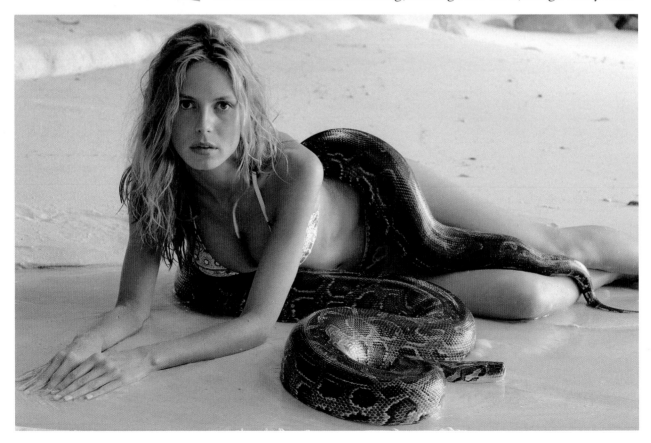

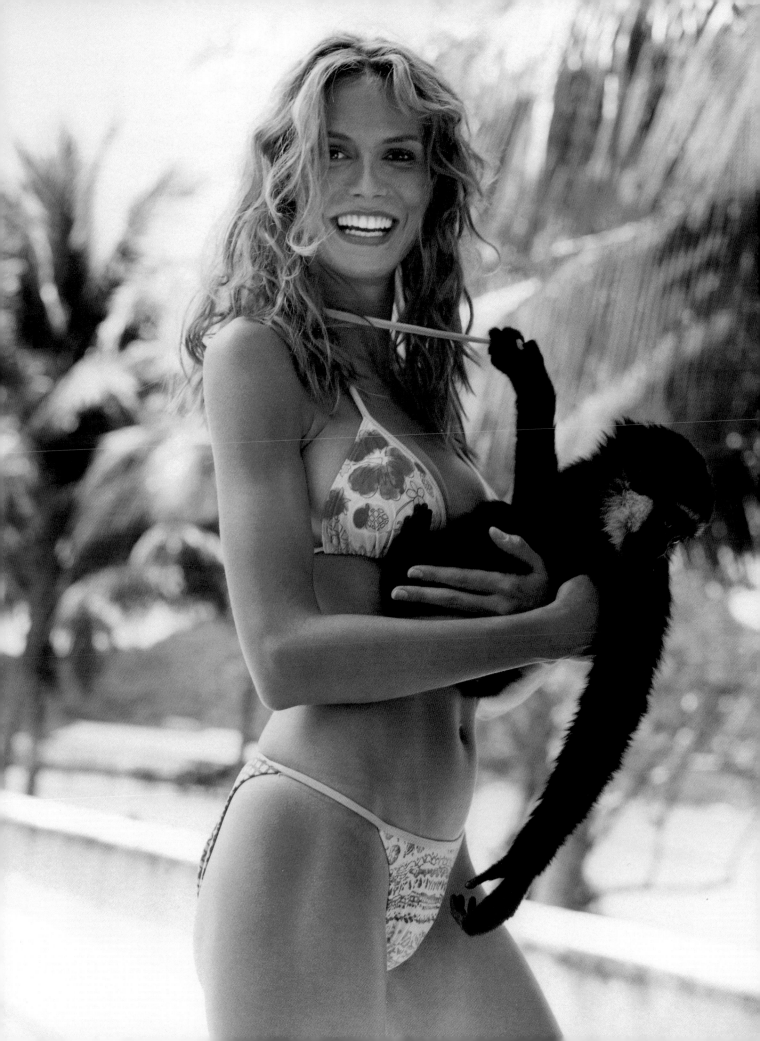

ing out over the presence of the enormous snake in their midst). I also shot a couple of rolls holding an adorable black monkey—adorable, that is, when the cheeky little thing wasn't pulling my hair out at the root or yanking off my bikini top.

While I wouldn't go so far as to say I endorse the saying "That which doesn't kill you makes you stronger," how about this:

That which doesn't challenge you makes you weaker.

Even if your job doesn't entail such exotic scenarios, it's nutritious for the spirit to try things that may seem (at first) weird or difficult. Because I'm passionate about travel (and because I passed the shark test), I'm hosting my own series of travel specials for Discovery Networks (their slogan: "Entertain Your Brain"). I always want to discover more about myself, and the only way that happens is if I expose my mind (and senses) to things it's unused to. In my TV specials, I want to cover the fun stuff (where to go shopping, how wine is made), but I also hope to convey a sense of what it's like to explore and savor another culture, and to show what a welcoming place the world can be.

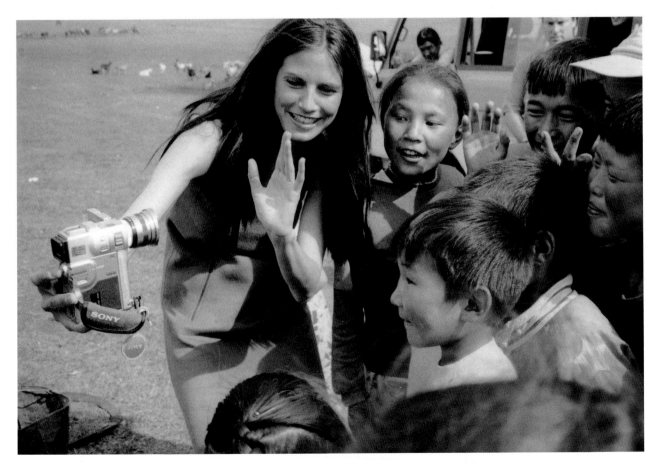

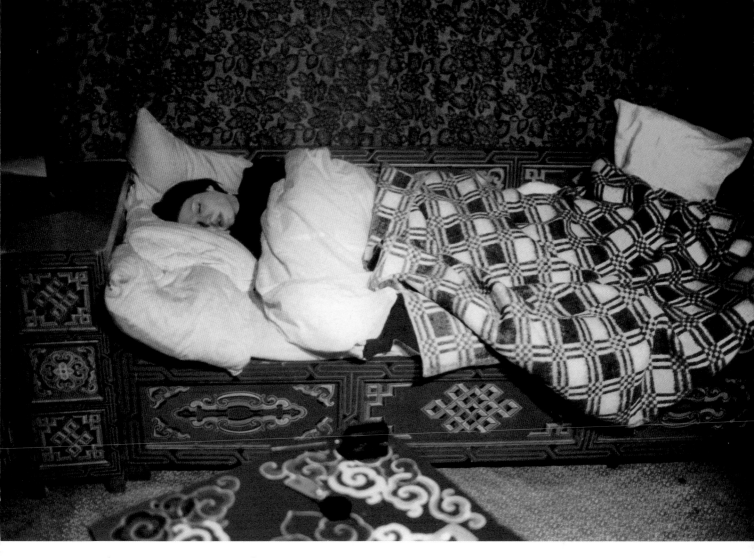

# make yourself more interesting . . . to others

By having new adventures, you become more interesting, hungrier to learn and do more, more confident that you can conquer what before had seemed daunting. While on assignment in Mongolia for *Marie Claire,* our jeep broke down, and we were stranded in the middle of nowhere for days. (The whole story? While driving through the Gobi Desert, our dilapidated fifteen-passenger van hit a man astride a horse. The horse and man were okay, but the van wouldn't budge and we were stuck in a spot that rarely saw signs of humanity.)

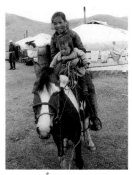

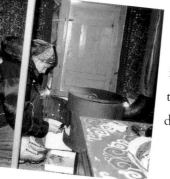

What did I take away from that experience? How resourceful people can be. How simple life can be. How you can subsist on very little, if that's all you have. When we finally made it to a nearby camp, instead of turning all prima donna, we slept in the tent where all the locals

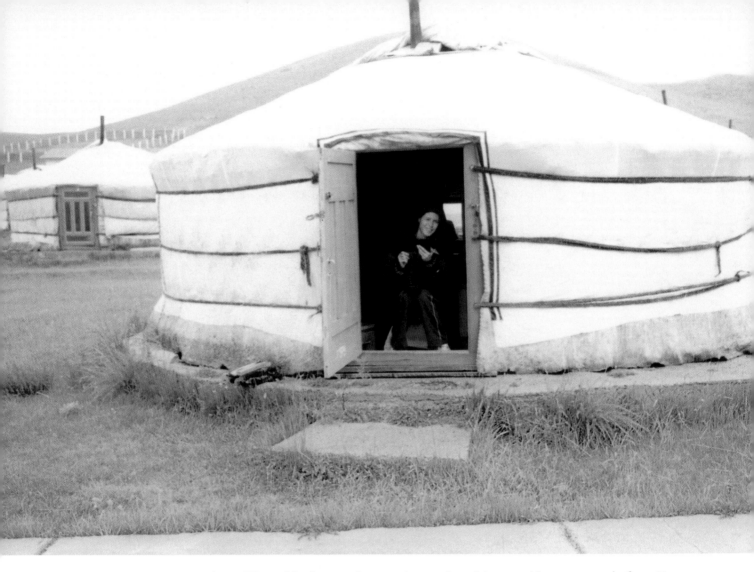

These yurts weren't exactly first-class accommodations (no one prepared us for the long walks to the loo, fermented horse milk, and the no-shower treatment), but the Mongolian nomads were so friendly and welcoming and the rolling hills of the countryside so beautiful, that Mongolia is a place I'll never forget.

slept. We trekked around every day, seeing things we'd never seen before. True, we subsisted mostly on *our* food—canned tuna fish and PowerBars—since fermented horse milk is an acquired taste. We attended the traditional Nadom athletic festival that featured bow-and-arrow competitions, wrestling, and horseback riding, a bit of sports theater that seemed closer to what I imagine the ancient Greek Olympics might have really been like than anything out there today.

By the end of the trip, Mongolia had become (and remains) one of my favorite places on Earth.

## wander woman

I'm on the road probably two thirds of the year. But I've always been comfortable with traveling because, when I was younger, my parents and brother and I often went camping, and as a child I'd been to Turkey, Italy, Yugoslavia, Hungary, and France.

I also thank my relatively modest upbringing—sharing a room with my brother; not being able to buy anything and everything I wanted—for making me more resourceful, a key attribute for a traveler.

The best way to see and get to know a new destination is to drive all over the place: That's how you put yourself in a position to encounter odd and wonderful things. (Early-morning runs or bike rides are also great for scouting the sights.) Ask the locals what to do and where to go, so you can take some time off the beaten path. But sometimes it's fun to do the touristy things, too. Recently, when I was in Egypt, we rode on camelback to the Great Pyramids, which were built by hand more than four thousand years ago, and marveled over the mummies and their treasures in the museum. It's a kick to feel like you're a character in some kind of history textbook, and it's humbling to recognize your place in the human timeline.

When it comes to eating, do as the natives do. In France, try the escargots, confit, foie gras, and tartare. In Japan, go to the authentic Japanese restaurants, and watch the sushi chefs at work or gamble on the blowfish. You needn't trek halfway around the world to eat at McDonald's. But for me, the key to having a good time?

**The Great Pyramids at sunrise on camelback . . . what could be more cliché? But sometimes the touristy stuff is the most fun of all.**

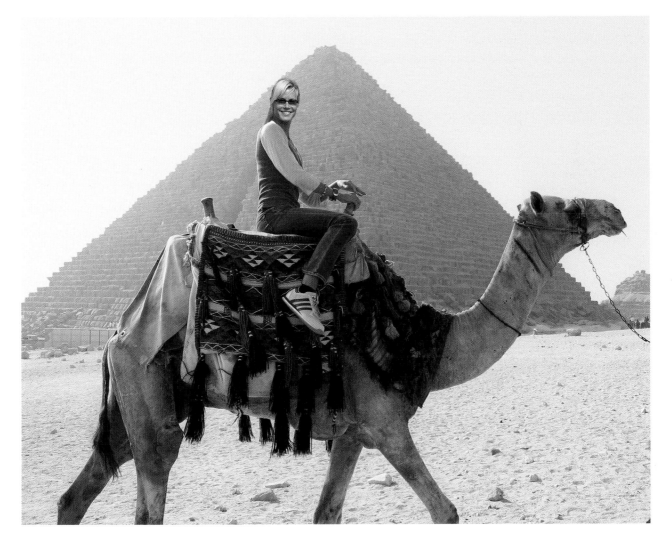

# my seven wonders of the world

I've been to lots of breathtaking, "the-postcard-doesn't-do-this-place-justice" destinations in my life, but these romantic, beautiful, and fascinating spots are among my all-time favorites:

**1. BALI.** I went to Bali for my honeymoon, thinking it would be all empty white beaches, sarongs, and flip-flops. It had all that but so much more. I was shocked at the diverse beauty of the island: the lush terraced rice fields with the mist lifting off them, the palaces and volcanoes, temples and crafts villages. You can smell paradise from the moment you get off the plane.

**2. THE TYROL.** Growing up, my family and I vacationed every winter in this Alpine region of northern Italy (bordering on Austria), and I dare you to name anything more wonderful than being stuck inside during a heavy mountain snow—you can't ski, you can't even get out, you're up so high that there's not much to do except drink hot chocolate and watch huge winter-wonderland flakes come down.

**3. PARIS.** It's glamorous and romantic, with those exquisite yellow limestone buildings bathed in light. I love sitting in cafés drinking café crème, watching the chic ladies pass by or discovering tiny, out-of-the-way patisseries and boutiques. The stores on the grand boulevards are incomparably stylish, but I always score something unique at the gigantic and historic flea markets on the outskirts of the city.

**4. THE AFRICAN SAVANNAH.** I've been on many safaris—in Kenya and in Tanzania—and it's such an overwhelming sensory experience, especially the natural music: Outside your tent at night you hear hippos munching on grass, hyenas laughing, lions prowling. The abundance of wildlife is surreal—I saw buffalo, elephants, giraffes, crocodiles, gazelle, a cheetah with five of her babies, and the (I was told) very rare sight of twelve lions eating a zebra, bloody carnage and all. One tip, learned at the Grumeti River: Never get between a hippo and the water.

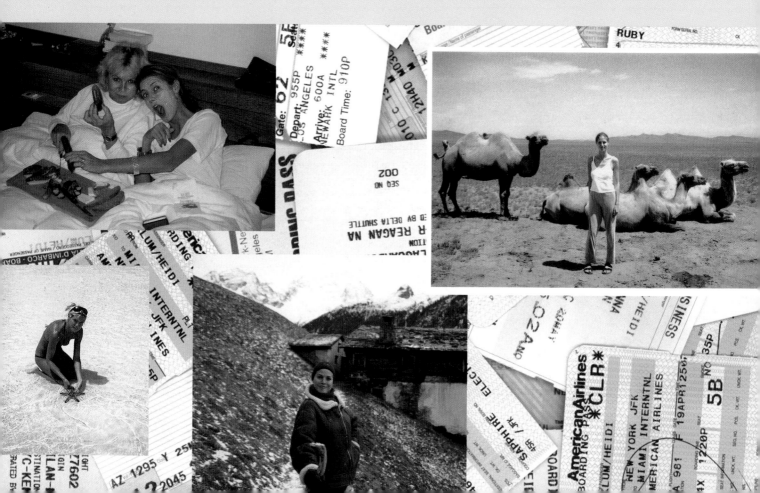

# (okay, so it's nine)

**5. HONG KONG.** The city still has a British-inspired elegance—the fancy old hotels, high tea service—but the underworld is what makes it riveting: pigs and chickens hanging in restaurant windows, not to mention some rather peculiar aphrodisiacs on the menu; at night, the lurid little alleys, the prostitutes publicly strutting their stuff, and nightclubs. The view from the peak of the city's gleaming high-rises is jawdropping, and the shopping (including huge jade and pearl markets) is overwhelming (in a good way). It's a modern bazaar.

**6. VENICE.** I love old things, so I fell hard for the city's ancient streets, old restaurants, rustic gondolas, endless history. Sure, they have Prada and Gucci and lots of modern chain stores and conveniences, but not everything there is straight and new and perfect, and you can find delights like stunning gold-leafed doges' palaces, frescoes, churches, masterworks of art, and antiques shops.

**7. THE MONGOLIAN DESERT.** There's nothing there. No cars, no congestion, no white noise, practically no trappings of civilization. And never has that word *trappings* seemed so apt. Almost nothing that seems to matter *here*—how you look, what brand you wear—matters there. The people could not be friendlier, and if you have a chance to stay in a yurt, do it.

**8. TOKYO.** It's so clean, chic, and sophisticated. The Japanese attention to detail is inspiring, from the elegant presentation of the food down to the heated toilet seat in my hotel (!). I couldn't stop studying the crazy outfits and hairstyles worn by the city's fashion-forward kids, and I was awed by the beautiful wooden temples and palaces.

**9. NEW YORK.** There's no place like it anywhere in the world—crazy, dirty streets giving rise to soaring silver office towers, European-style cafés and shops in SoHo contrasting with the wide, elegant boulevards of the Upper East Side. From the yellow cabs and 24/7 delivery options to the melting-pot citizenry and New Yorkers' brusque, efficient energy, it's my kind of city, my kind of home. Right now, it *is* home.

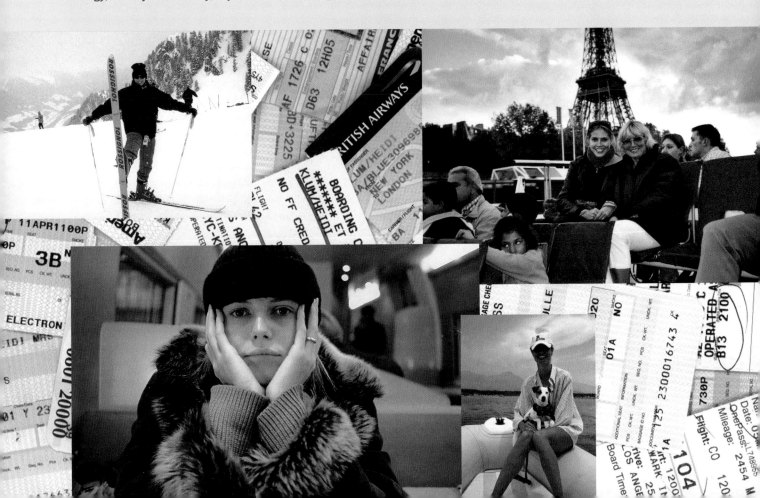

I've flown to certain places I was hardly keen to go to (though part of my lack of enthusiasm can always be traced to being trapped on a plane), but I'll always make myself think of the positive part of what's to come: Every spot in the world has something about it that sticks with me and compels me to return.

## make every trip a journey

*While traveling, be productive.* Everyone feels so guilty when they're away—all that work piling up, the unreturned phone calls—that it can take away some of the sting if you plan to accomplish something modest but precise in those hours when you're captive (like on a plane). When I fly, I sometimes doodle designs or read a script. Most important, I always make a huge "to do" list of all that I need to take care of when I return from my trip—everything from arranging vet appointments to work-

### DON'T BE A PACK RAT

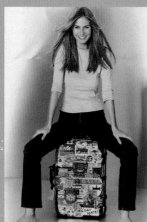

For ten years (and counting), there's one companion I will not travel without: my Samsonite hard case, covered with stickers from all over the world.

➤ People often suggest bringing things—a favorite pillow or candles—to personalize your hotel room and make yourself feel cozy, but I'm a minimalist. Try not to carry your entire home with you; otherwise, you might as well just stay there.

➤ For up to a week, I bring two cute outfits—a little black dress and a nice pair of jeans, maybe a jean jacket (which you can wear with the black dress). They all adapt nicely to dressy or casual situations. I also stuff in a great purse, shoes that go with both outfits, and a wrap that can be worn with anything.

➤ For makeup, I forgo all the colors and steps and just pack a little bag with bare necessities: gloss, lipstick, concealer, sunscreen, and mascara.

➤ Don't forget those adapters for international outlets!

➤ I love to anticipate serendipity, so I leave room in my suitcase for new purchases . . . or I pack an empty bag or knapsack. (If I buy a lot of clothes and there's no room in my bag, I just wear lots of layers on the flight back.) The combo of suitcase-bursting-at-seams and stern-looking-suspicious-customs-officer makes for an unpleasant reentry.

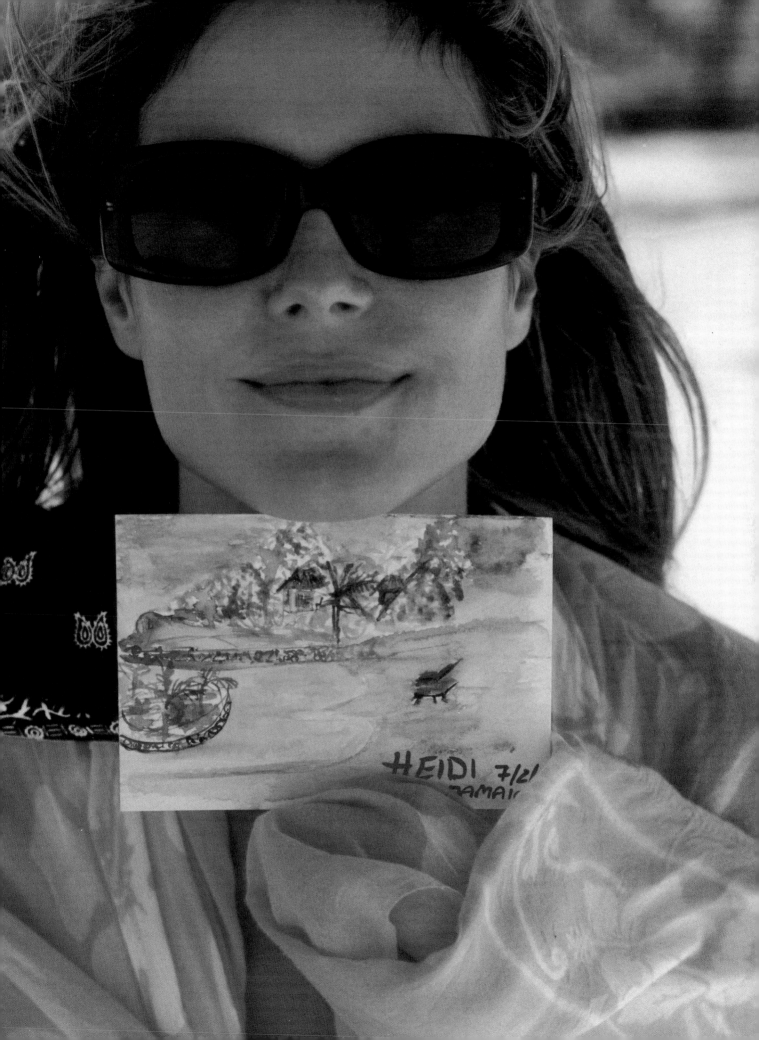

ing on a certain overdue book! That way, it's fresh in my mind while I'm still in active mode but I can let it go and enjoy my vacation once I've written it down and organized my thoughts and action plans.

*The trip starts as soon as you step off the plane.* We tend to brace ourselves for the tedium of getting from the point of disembarkation (to use the lovely word on those little airplane cards you have to fill out) to the hotel, so it becomes hard to enjoy the fact that we're *already* in new surroundings. Every minute you're away counts—and given that you may spend hours each way getting to and from the airport or train station, appreciate the time for what it is. Look around, take pictures, get oriented.

*Pamper yourself when you get there.* The first thing I do when I check in to a hotel—after calling my mother to tell her I've arrived in one piece—is take a bath. A good soak after a long flight not only feels incredible, but it brings on drowsiness and helps you avoid jet lag.

*Send postcards.* I always send them to friends and family—my mother's kitchen is full of postcards of every place I've been to, some of which I've painted myself. In this age of Internet e-mail and chat, there's a quaint pleasure in knowing you've sent a friend an actual piece of writing.

*Book your activities locally.* Travel agents and package deals provide a sense of security before you go, but the locals are bound to be more knowledgeable. Hotel or resort staff can help you with your itinerary or local activities, and their information will be more current (weather changes, unexpected developments, etc.). Concierges can recommend reputable guides, locations, and modes of transport.

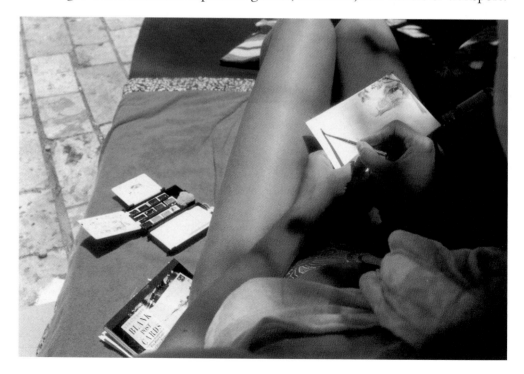

# HOW TO TAKE BEAUTIFUL TRAVEL PHOTOS
BY GILLES BENSIMON, PHOTOGRAPHER AND PUBLICATION DIRECTOR OF *ELLE* USA

*I've worked with Gilles dozens of times, and what I love about his photos is the way he brings out my personality and isn't afraid to print a goofy candid picture. When we're on location, he's always snapping photos of flowers or sites or other things that catch his eye.*

First, remember that taking pictures is a very special act, despite the fact that photography has become so common, even disposable. Pictures bring memories to life; you don't realize just how evocative they will be in a few years.

Because photography is so special, the moment that you capture in a picture has to mean something. I'm not against taking pictures of someone standing in front of the Statue of Liberty or on the Champs-Elysées; it can help you keep a record of your life. But try to convey the feeling of a unique or vanishing moment. What I love in photography, even fashion photography, is my awareness that the moment I'm trying to document is never going to occur

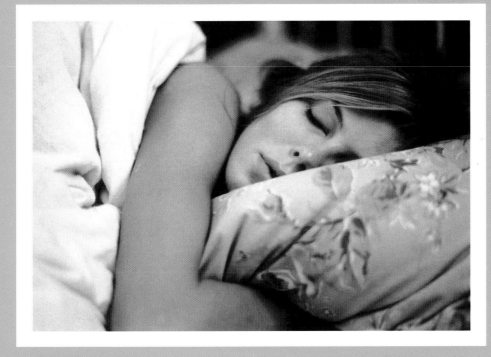

again. In that way, I believe photography is really on some level about death, or the passage of time.

How to capture that evanescence? It's easy. Photograph everything that you have a feeling for: the road unfolding in front of your dashboard or the clouds suspended beyond the airplane's wing; the remains on the plate of a great meal; rumpled bedsheets or your lover's body while he or she is sleeping; a sunset; two strangers talking; a crowd of people at a wedding; a dirty ashtray.

You just can't plan that image too far in advance. You need to be clever and sneak up on it (though you should ask others if it's all right to take their picture). Sometimes I shoot a lot of pictures in succession in order to get those one or two images that perfectly describe the movement, and the essence, of a subject. Try to bring out the detail of what you're photographing by moving a few steps closer. Otherwise you'll just see a little head or object floating against a flat background. You can never be too close.

I prefer to get my film printed on paper with a white border, which frames the image nicely. However, I don't like to process my personal film right away when I get back from a trip. That way, a few weeks or even months later, I get the film back and the images I've caught are a total surprise.

All photographs are good. If you take lots of them, you'll be amazed by just how talented you really are.

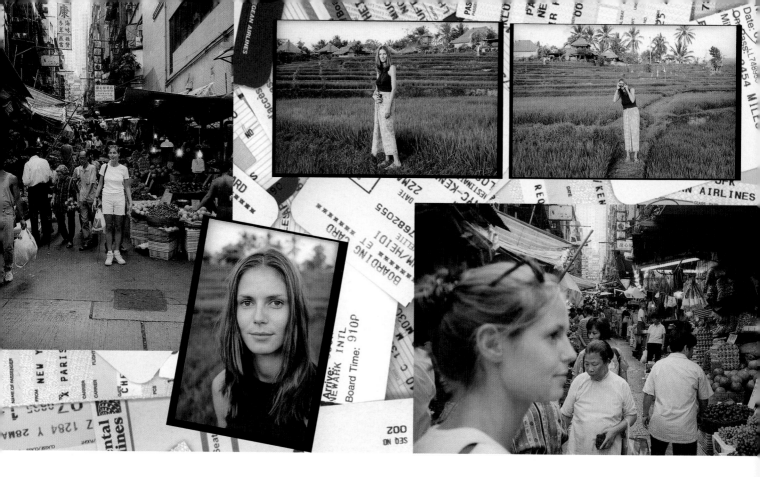

*Never just think "photo op."* Standing before the Taj Mahal, you can't believe what a stunning picture it will make. But it's not enough just to snap a roll, check out the guidebook, and move on. Try to find some off-the-beaten-track places, and enjoy those as well.

Travel allows you experiences that are not possible in your day-to-day life. It may be a cliché, but

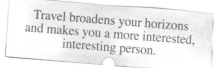

Travel broadens your horizons and makes you a more interested, interesting person.

That's the real payoff. We all have something that scares us but that we've secretly always wanted to do . . . so get on a plane, train, or automobile (even a camel or elephant), and get to some locale that isn't right around the corner. Having screwed up the courage to dive into a circle of Caribbean reef sharks—that's something I'll never forget. More important, it's something that forever after strengthened me, so the benefits of that adventure stay with me every day. So think of me when you're eating that bizarre delicacy or hiking to a jaw-dropping vista or chatting (with lots of hand gestures) to a bemused local—and hey: Remember to drop a postcard!

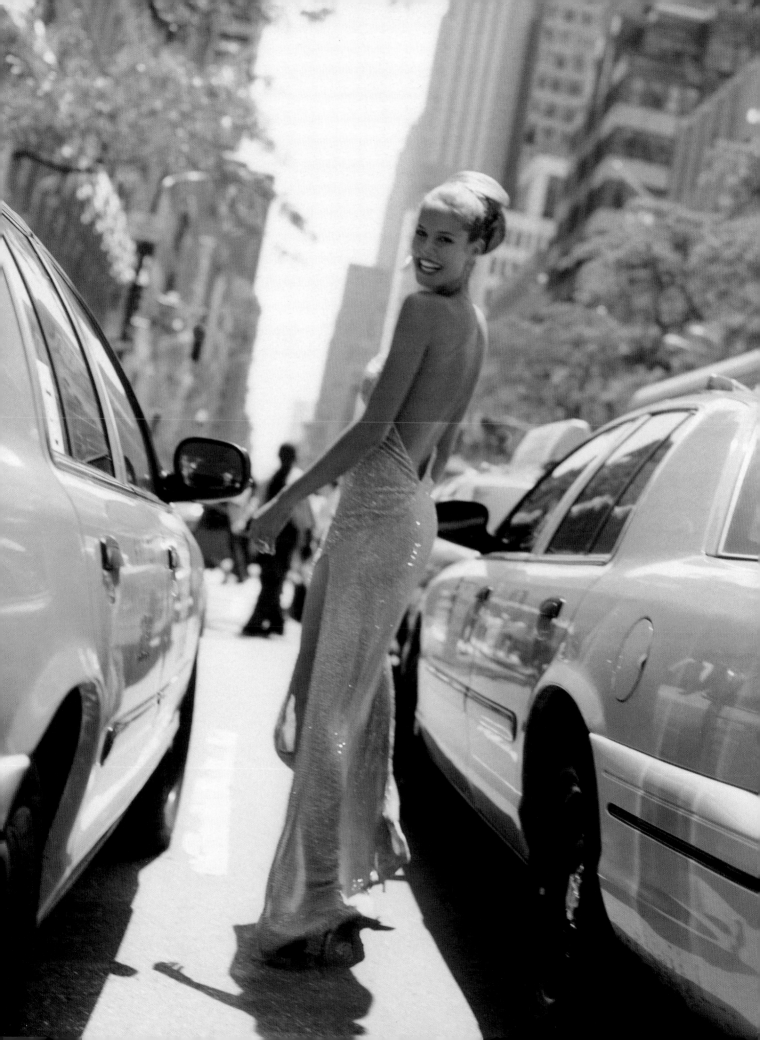

# FUN

**RULE 8**

*have a* blast
while it lasts

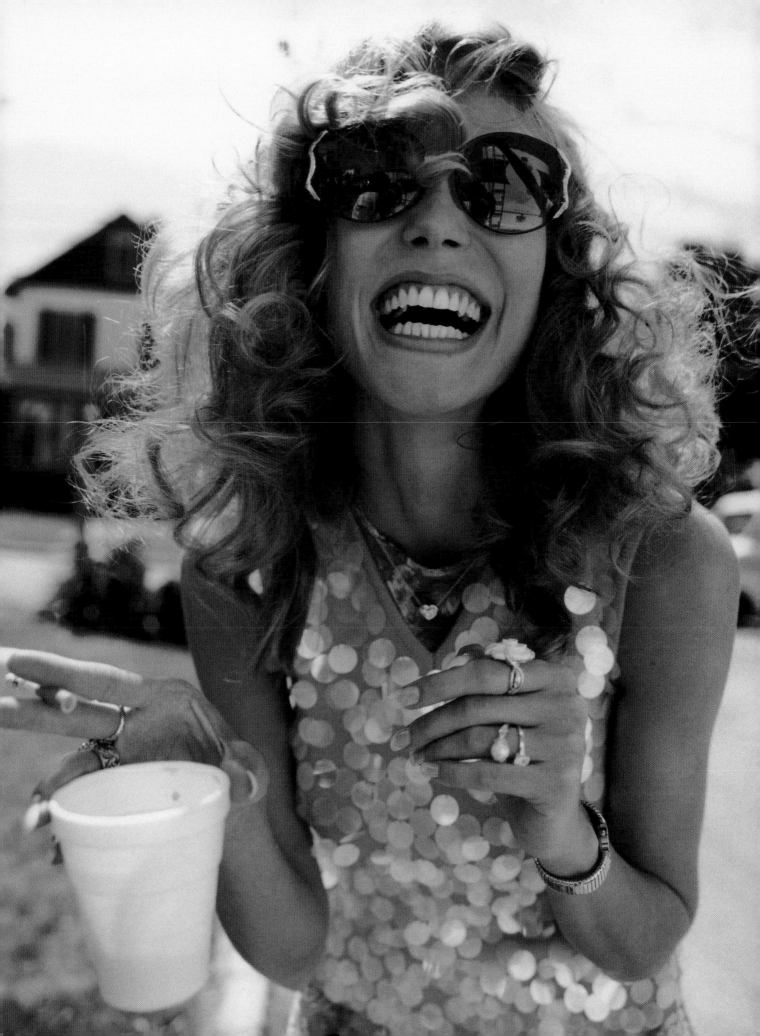

Unlike most professions—accounting, say, or medicine—a model's career is rather abbreviated. If you were discovered "late" (e.g., after twenty), that clock is always ticking a little too loudly for comfort. That's why, for the duration of the time that I'm privileged to have the job that I do, I always want to approach it with the right attitude. Part of that is making the best of every situation and trying to have as much fun as possible.

When I'm on a photo shoot, I'm working, sure, but it's hardly drudgery. There's almost always a boom box blasting something really catchy to help us get in the mood. By "us" I don't mean just the models, but everyone—photographers, assistants, stylists, makeup artists. And where there's music, there's singing. And dancing.

All that positive energy makes the experience more fun. Positivity is an attitude I keep in mind not just when I'm working, but also when I'm doing almost anything, even routine (*especially* routine); after all, it's better for you, not to mention your health, to get a positive buzz out of *any* experience, rather than just go through the motions. Driving in traffic becomes a jam session when I'm blasting music at ear-splitting volumes. Even vacuuming—that's right, *vacuuming*—can be more fun by making it about something other than cleaning. Ever consider using that typically dreary chore as a way to break in a fabulous new pair of shoes? You feel as if you're accomplishing something besides sucking up dust balls.

With a little creativity, anything (well almost) can be fun.

I know that not everyone can do their job while blasting a boom box. When we're modeling, the days can be very long and physically exhausting (I might have to hold one position to the point where my muscles shake, and we sometimes wait endlessly between setups for shots), but we're not exactly doing brain surgery or teaching first graders. We're hoping to create beautiful images, so we try to entertain ourselves while doing it. From one shoot to the next, I'm often working with many of the same crew, so we grow familiar with one another and become this instant, random family. The talk is gossipy and frivolous (who's dating whom . . . who broke up with whom . . . how constipated we are . . . details of

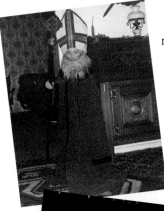

recent sexploits . . . ). Okay, maybe it's a little more outrageous than six co-workers standing around a water cooler, but I always try to remember that it's the people you work with who make the experience great (or not), so it's important to try to get along.

This is especially important on location shoots, when we may all be stranded together on some South Pacific island or remote mountaintop. Once we lose our light (modeling schedules are much more dependent on the sun's movement than on the hands of a clock, which is why we often start our days in the dark), we'll all go a little nuts—sing around a bonfire or go out to local bars and clubs (if there are any) for karaoke, dancing, and drinking. The last night of the shoot is the wildest, because we don't have to look particularly fresh the next day. I remember a shoot on St. Barth's, where the hairstylist, Italo, cooked for us every day (he's been known to transport his pasta machine halfway around the globe), and on the final night someone put on striptease music and we all did a classic burlesque bump and grind.

Despite the fun I have doing my job, I'm not a party girl. Although I love dressing up and going out—I attend lots of events—you won't catch me dancing on the table at some club. I'm certainly not one of those Beautiful People types who will actually *fly* to another city if there's a big party going on there.

So how did I become, in the last few years, the host and mastermind of what I think is fair to call one of New York City's most exciting parties of the year?

# it's my party . . .

My annual Halloween fête—an A-list (if I may say so) party that attracts hundreds of people, all in wild costume, to a cool and unusual venue each October 31—didn't come about because I desperately needed one more event to go to. (If you're a model in New York City, one thing you do *not* lack for is invitations.) It happened because I just adore theme parties.

I have fond childhood memories of my girlfriends coming over and of my father helping to orchestrate all these diversions: egg-walking, potato-sack races, musical chairs, speed eating. I even loved to play math games, in which Dad would rattle off a bunch of math problems (*"Take x . . . double it . . . minus this . . . "*) and we'd try to come up with the right answer. When

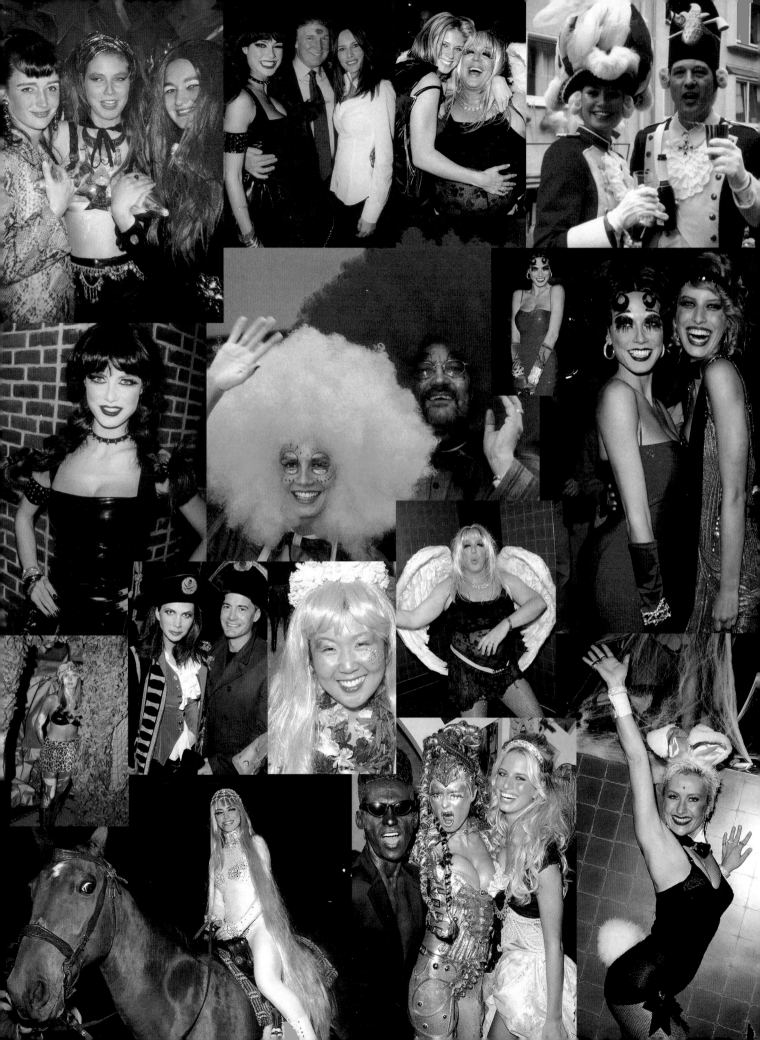

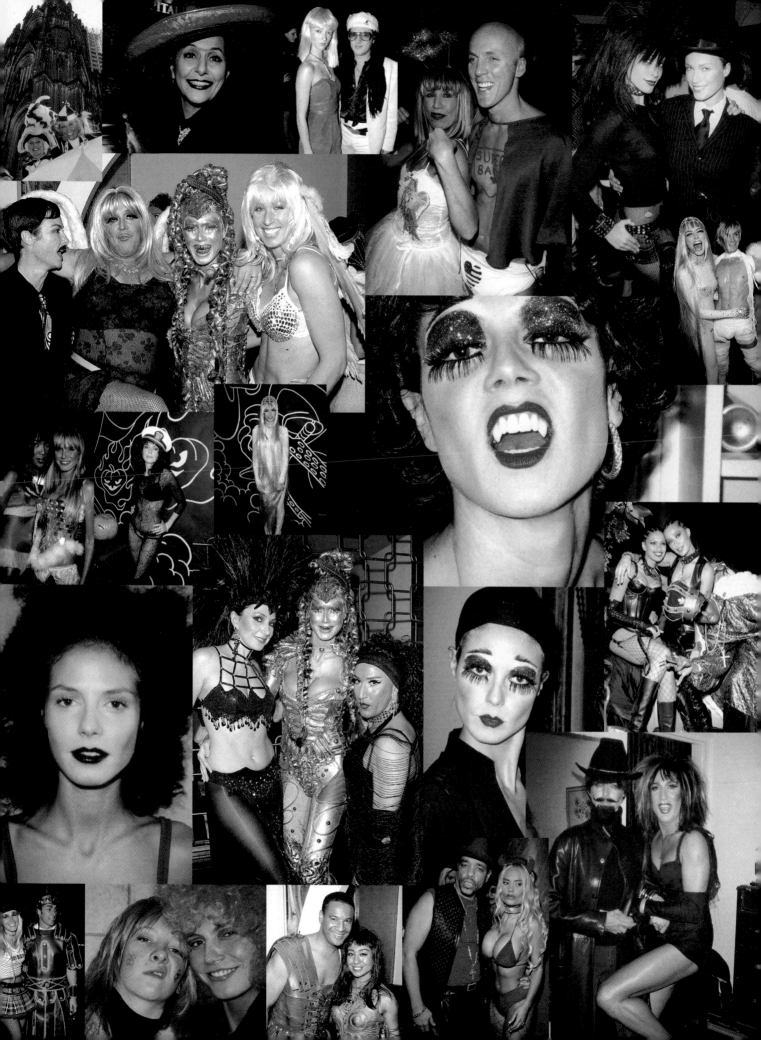

I got older, we used to do themed birthdays; one year we were all aliens from outer space, the next we were the Flintstones.

I'm nostalgic for these scenes not so much because they were parties but because they all shared an aspect of make-believe—a carnivalesque atmosphere where you could play at being something or someone else. It's no wonder I love Halloween, the ultimate dressing-up holiday. Several years ago, I noticed how lots of my New York friends—lots of New Yorkers, in general—never wanted to dress in costume, to get out of their own skins for one night. (Was it just too corny? Too uncool?) I went to so many parties where it was the same old thing each time—everyone dancing, listening to music, drinking the latest apple/peppermint/sake martini and trying to have a conversation—so I thought it was time to mix things up a little. Besides, I think dressing up changes people, lets their imaginations run wild. (Isn't that the principle the fashion industry is built on?)

So I decided to throw a hard-core Halloween party where costumes were not "optional." I always get excited about planning my own outfit, and I start sketch-

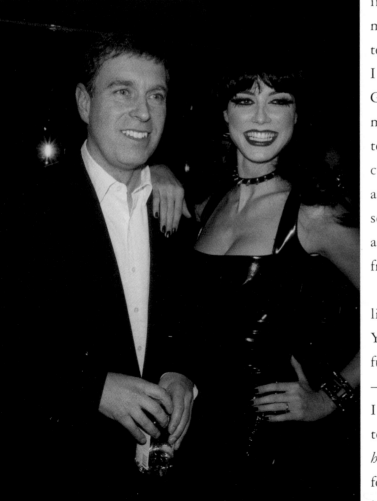

I gave Prince Andrew quite a scare when I tried to kiss him on the forehead to jazz up his (nonexistent) Halloween costume. I just wanted to see if he would turn into a frog!

ing it out weeks in advance. I like to make a big statement with an over-the-top get-up, so I'm no longer recognizable. I have gone as, among others, Lady Godiva riding on a white horse (one of the more challenging guests I've ever brought to a party), Betty Boop, for which I got a custom-made figure with cartoon curves, and a gold-painted space alien (silver just seemed so unoriginal), complete with actual gold teeth that I commissioned from a dentist who works with rappers.

At first, people thought my party was like most other costume parties in New York—Yeah, sure, whatever, I'll wear a funny hat or put some glitter on my face—but eventually they got the point that I was serious. And once everyone started to treat it like a costume party *where you had to come in costume,* it not only transformed the mood of the whole night, but it also became a kind of Can-You-Top-

This? game, with more and more people wearing increasingly outrageous get-ups.

The Duke of York—aka Prince Andrew—apparently didn't understand my ground rules. When he showed up (I didn't know he was coming) with Donald Trump one year, he looked like . . . the Duke of York. No disguise, nothing. Hadn't even dyed his hair purple. When we were introduced, I challenged him. "Well?" I asked. "Where's your costume?" He just sort of shrugged.

Our exchange got a lot of coverage for another reason: Here's me, dressed as "Heidi Ho"—a rather unsavory version of the Austrian lass of the mountains, clad in black leather, studs, and buckles—standing face-to-face with the second son of the Queen of England. After I'd dressed him down (in a manner of speaking) about not bothering to suit up, I leaned toward him, about to give him a big red-lipstick kiss on his forehead. "I don't think that's such a good idea," he said. Although I *didn't* kiss him, the very close encounter was photographed, splashed all over the pages of the British tabloids, and blown way out of proportion.

The most outrageous party I've ever been to (aside from my own) is the *Vanity Fair* Oscar party. It seems as if every famous entertainer you know from past and present is there: all these iconic actors and actresses and musicians, along with the flavors-of-the-month. Everyone's decked out—wearing the most fabulous dresses, the most overstyled hair, the most exquisite and expensive jewels. They all look great, if a little surreal. There's Jack Nicholson, cooling his heels over by the bar! And Meryl Streep looking like all of the characters she's ever played at once, luminous and poised. After all, an entire industry—an entire city, guys included—has, like me, spent most of that day sitting under a blow-dryer.

At events like these, I still feel like Cinderella at the ball, in awe of all the talent (I still get so starstruck that I ask celebrities if I can get a picture of myself with them for my scrapbook) and the opulent surroundings—but not least because by the end of the night, I have to give up the borrowed dress and jewels. So I try to enjoy every minute of my night as a princess, driving to the ceremony with my publicist Desirée and a few of our friends, for instance, and letting everyone take turns wearing the $15 million yellow diamond necklace that I borrowed from David Orgell. (Yes, I returned it intact before my limo turned into a pumpkin and my dress into sweatpants.)

Going to these kinds of circuses is undeniably fun, but my real social fix is satisfied by dinner parties with friends. When it works (and it usually does), that kind of evening has, in its way, everything that my Halloween party does: Everyone shows up. All the people you want to see are there. Everyone has fun, and no one wants to go home.

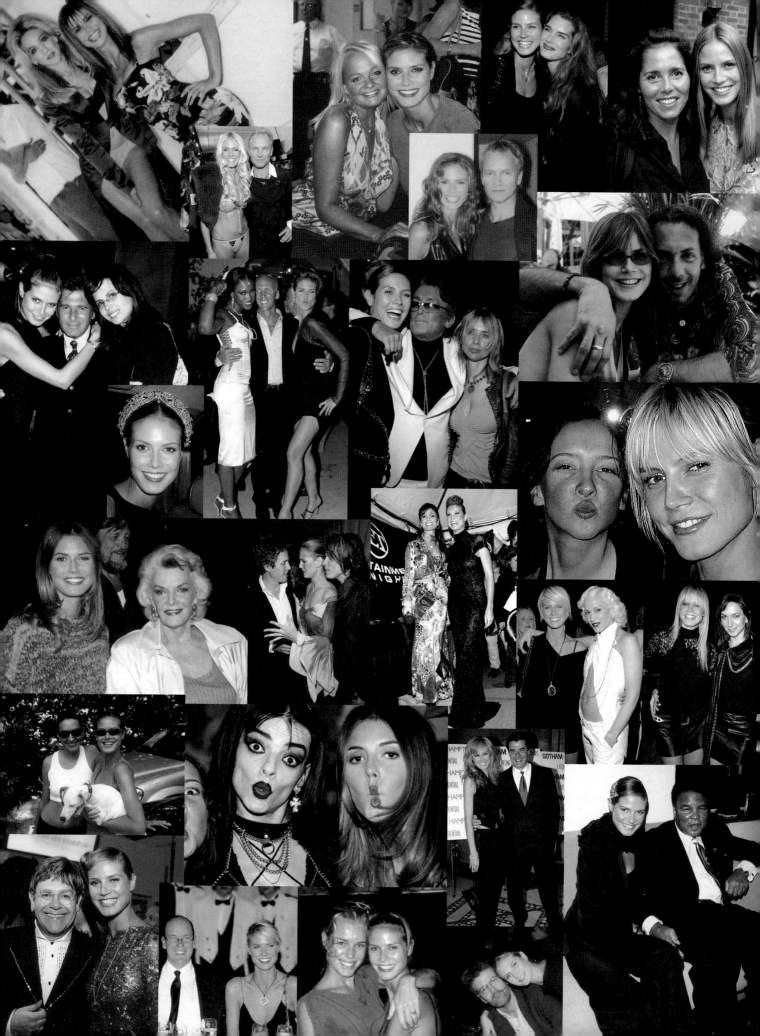

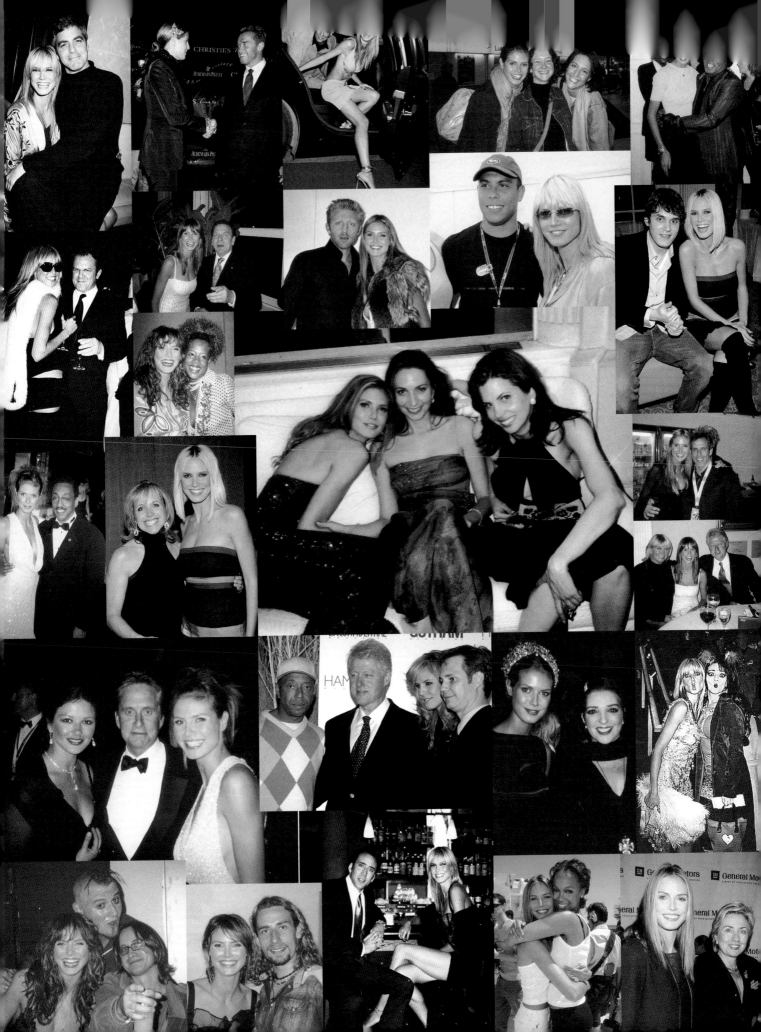

# friendship on the fly

I come in contact with lots and lots of people, some famous, most not. I have been asked how I know who's really my friend, and who just wants something from me. To me it's pretty obvious. Do you love being with a person, or don't you? When I'm home in Germany, I still hang out with my two oldest friends, Karin and Nina. (Sometimes I'll bring one of them as my date to an event, and we have fun rummaging through my closet looking for something for her to wear.) Even if I'm halfway around the world, we're always calling or e-mailing one another, offering advice on the other's career or love life, so we never go for long stretches without being in touch.

At a certain age, however, it can be a challenge to make new friends you really feel close to, no matter how public a life you lead. It's so easy to get distracted by responsibility and obligations—jobs, travel, romantic relationships—that it can seem at times as if we don't even need friends. Of course, nothing could be further from the truth. Not surprisingly, some of my best friends are those I've made through work—my publicist, a fashion stylist, a photographer's assistant. You end up being thrown together again and again, and eventually you gel, or you don't. You can always tell who the insincere ones are, because they never try to get a sense of who you really are; they just want to know about your work and who else you hang out with.

Because the road can be such a lonely place (say what you want about first-class airport lounges, they don't hold a candle to a friend's living room), I definitely relish what little time I do get with the people I love to hang out with. Tyra Banks and I live in different cities, but when we have the good fortune to fly somewhere together for a photo shoot, we start our own little reunion party in the front of the plane. Tyra

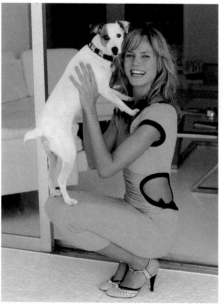

likes to bring her own food on board—a very pungent kind of soul food, which she kindly shares with me (we annoy the flight attendants by refusing all offers of bread or desserts—such typical models!). Then we spend the next several hours yapping away about our latest ventures, guys, sex, gossip about the agencies, you name it. We don't get to see each other all that often, but when we do, it's always real.

I always go out of my way to be friendly to people I meet, and every once in a while one of those encounters blossoms into a friendship. Fortunately, I now have pals in many parts of the world, so I have dozens of international numbers programmed into my cell phone and there are lots of places I visit where I can be assured of having company when exploring a city, rather than confining myself to my hotel room watching pay-per-view and ordering room service.

## MUSIC FOR EVERY OCCASION

BY ANTHONY KIEDIS, LEAD SINGER, RED HOT CHILI PEPPERS

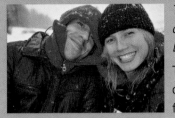

*The first time I laid eyes on Anthony . . . let's just say I couldn't take them off of him. Since then, he's taught me so much about music—old and new—so who better to help you come up with a soundtrack to your life?*

The funny thing about listening to music for a certain occasion is that it keeps changing. A song or a record that tore my heart out and connected me to the loving force of the universe three months ago might not ever do the same again. It's a constant and evolving search . . . and therein lies the beauty and the adventure of sound. It's abstract and infinite while working like god-given holistic medicine, affecting each ear in a unique way.

1. If you should ever find yourself driving northbound on the 101, headed for a Big Sur surf trip with two of your favorite allies, just pop the Germs (GI) into your player. Invigorating tendencies will erupt from your core.

2. Blonde Redhead made a record called *La Mia Vita Violenta,* which sounds so magical while taking a morning shower. Not to get all sexual right off the bat, but it does lend itself to those feelings.

3. If you ever feel like too many days have passed without any dancing, just pop in *James Brown Live at the Apollo.* Ass-shaking blood flow is sure to follow.

4. Dolly Parton wrote and recorded a song called "I Will Always Love You" in 1974. If you want to sit in the dark and cry about how much you used to be in love with someone, this is the prescription. After you have drained yourself of tears and heartbreak, play the 1973 recording of her song "Jolene." Picks me up every time.

5. Music to get dressed to: Ramones. Their first record gets me in the mood for any high- or low-powered outing into the night. Reminds me not to take myself too seriously. Life is but a dream, so why not invite the Ramones?

6. Feel like getting away from everything pretentious and full of shit? Play Fela and Afrika 70. The record is called *Zombie.* This music from the Nigerian superhero cleans the spirit and shows us how to move.

7. On hot summer nights driving around Los Angeles with my moon roof open, I'm mighty inclined to listen to David Bowie's *Young Americans.* It reminds me of my childhood in the seventies and makes me feel emotionally strong. Strong like I could write songs and deep kiss my girl.

8. Simple things seem to stand the test of time. Marc Bolan wrote some of the most enduring, simple, classic, perfect songs ever and put them on a record called *The Slider.* Special occasion not required.

9. My friend John and I shared a bus on our tour last year. We would listen religiously to Nick Drake's *Bryter Layter,* just sitting there in the dark smiling and driving through nighttime places like New Mexico.

10. Number 10 is for the hundreds of other pieces of music I hope we can all hunt down in our quest for happiness. God Bless, and until we meet again . . .

# find your bliss

Obviously I'm a big cheerleader of finding pleasure in all aspects of life—working, eating, driving, flying on an airplane—but I also think it helps to have passion for certain activities that are *meant* to be fun. I'm talking about hobbies, whatever they

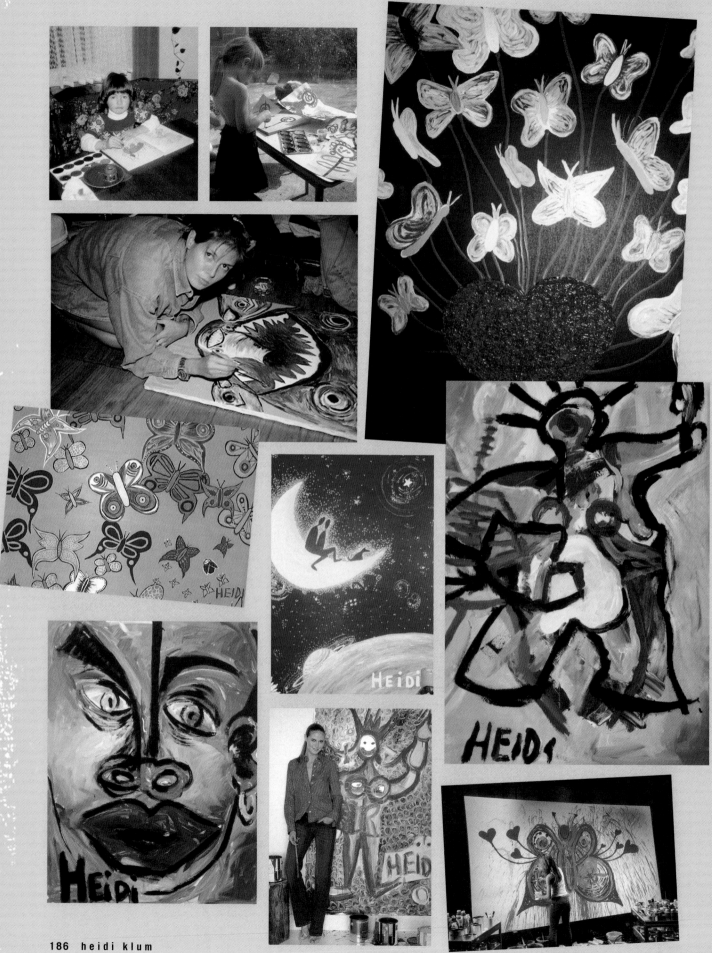

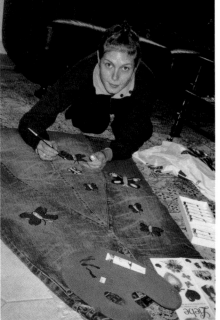

You have to take time to do the things you love. Here I am painting a skirt for charity—and someone actually bought it!

may be. Me, I love to cook, to shop—every Sunday, I hit my local flea market. Hobbies make you a more interesting person to yourself and to others.

Of all my diversions, probably the one I care most about is art. I love to paint—from big juicy oil paintings to postcard-sized watercolors (I have a wallet-sized paint kit that's easy to travel with). I have no real formal training in it; I just paint what moves me, and I keep painting until I think it's done. Maybe I'll do a huge red heart to show my love for someone, or a fish for a friend who has an aquarium. I especially like giving art to friends as gifts: My friend the fish-lover was ecstatic (I hope!) when she got the giant painting that was meant to stand behind her tank where the fish could see it; my grandmother, then in the hospital for an operation, was cheered by the green canvas teeming with butterflies that I'd made. Often, too, I'll go to a local pottery studio and paint mugs, vases, and frames to give as gifts.

The process of painting is personal, the result is unique, and it's a labor of love. (Although it's not always successful. Perhaps my boldest art experiment—covering my naked body in paint, then rolling around on the canvas—turned out to be just a big wet blotch; not quite the sophisticated abstract expression I'd envisioned.) Who cares if your crafts don't turn out to be Martha Stewart perfect?

Whenever possible, I try to turn occasions into events—whether it's waxing Jay Leno's legs onstage, or making a giant party out of a little girl's lasting wish still to play dress-up. Maybe it sounds a little flamboyant, but to me, being a fun-seeker shows that you're open to all possibilities, that you want to make life as full as you can. Why *wouldn't* you try to suck as much joy as you can out of each moment?

Romantically, I find there's nothing more unattractive than a person who doesn't have their "own thing" but just takes on your life, and nothing is more attractive than someone who has many passions they call their own, want to talk about, want to show and share with you. And the beautiful part is, you don't have to be a genius at any of it to make it worthwhile! You just need to make it yours to care about it and to enjoy it.

Isn't that what makes for a good adventure?

Good sex?

A good job?

A good life?

You should take your work seriously and your fun seriously. Work hard, play hard. Otherwise, what's the point?

# HAVING A GO AT THE WORLD

BY BONO, LEAD SINGER OF U2

*I love Bono's voice, and his lyrics are not just beautiful but have that rare quality in music: They're meaningful. He's mysterious and a little shy—guess that explains those tinted glasses. But he's also a great observer and very curious about the world—and, as everyone knows, he's committed to doing his part to improve it. Here's what he says about how anyone can have an impact.*

Rock stars, if they're honest, have two instincts: They want to have fun, and they want to change the world. If they didn't want to make an impression, they'd have picked a quieter calling . . . carpentry, hand weaving, pottery (though Grayson Perry has changed all that). Here are five points to remember, if you want to have a go at the world.

**1.** Things don't have to be as they are. You don't have to be as you were. The world is more malleable than you think, more elastic. It is not all set in concrete and where it is, at least stick your fingers in before it dries.

**2.** Vote. In the history of men, women, and civilization, democracy is the freak . . . a meager blip in ten thousand years of living under tyrannies of one kind or another. It's an amazing thing. Use it or you'll lose it, sure as anything.

**3.** Remember—your local politicians are working for you. You're paying their wages. Annoy them; they read their mail.

**4.** You are where you shop. Become label, not brand conscious (i.e., what's on the label, where it was made, who made it, and what it's made from). The apparel business in particular is often scandalous in its disregard for all of the above. Child labor in sweatshops, toxic dyes, etc. Read *Cradle to Cradle* by William McDonough.

**5.** Do not bore the arse off your friends. In fact, make friends in unexpected places. Politicians are not afraid of rock stars and student activists. They're much more nervous about church folk and soccer moms. The thing that really terrifies them is when rock stars and student activists start hanging out with church folk and soccer moms.

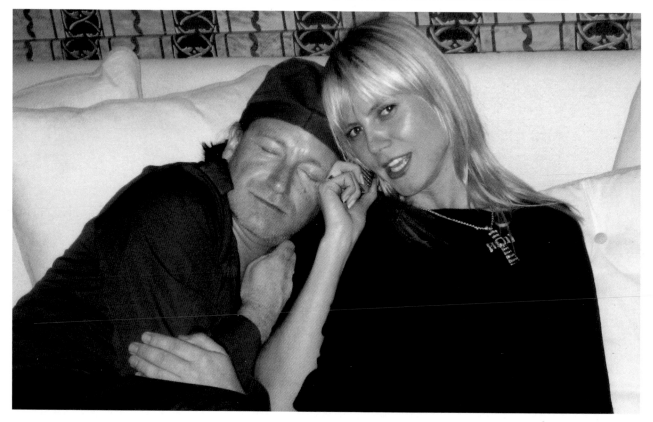

# one more thing

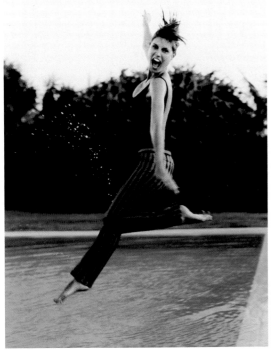

I hope that some of these anecdotes and ideas and tips will inspire you to try to become the person that you always envisioned yourself to be. Through perseverence, hard work, and a little bit of luck, I've been able to achieve a good many of those dreams that I dreamed as a young girl in Germany.

But it's important to stress that I couldn't have attained these goals on my own. If you think about it, if it weren't for my parents nurturing my adventurous spirit, I might still be living in my little village, never having the courage to pursue the things that meant the most to me.

But developing a never-say-die, try-anything-once spirit isn't enough to get you to the pinnacle you seek. It seems to me that probably the most important key to getting what you want in this life—and this takes both humility and smarts—is acknowledging what you don't know and seeking out trustworthy people who do. I've talked a lot about the advice I get from others, and that's a huge aspect of my life and growth. I've surrounded myself with a team I can count on, to offer not only professional advice but support, friendship, different perspectives, and complementary strengths. Who's part of Team Heidi? Family, friends, agents, publicists, bookers, attorneys, trainers, beauty and health gurus—uh oh . . . I think I've waded into diva territory here.

But here's the takeaway (and even if you're in a profession that doesn't require so many sorts of advisers, it doesn't matter, because the fundamental principle's the same):

> The more brains you have on your side, the better.

It doesn't have to be people you're paying; you can ask a bunch of friends to help. In return, you can offer your help in your particular area of expertise. No one reaches their goals or, more important, enjoys a happy, fulfilling life, without the support of those near and dear, people who care about you as a person rather than what you can do for them; people who have your back in any situation. Sure, you have to be your own boss. Yes, I want to know what agreements I've entered into, and I don't want to leave final decisions to lawyers and agents. But, however you do it, gather around you a team that's smart, savvy, and compassionate, and there's very little that can stop you from reaching your dreams.

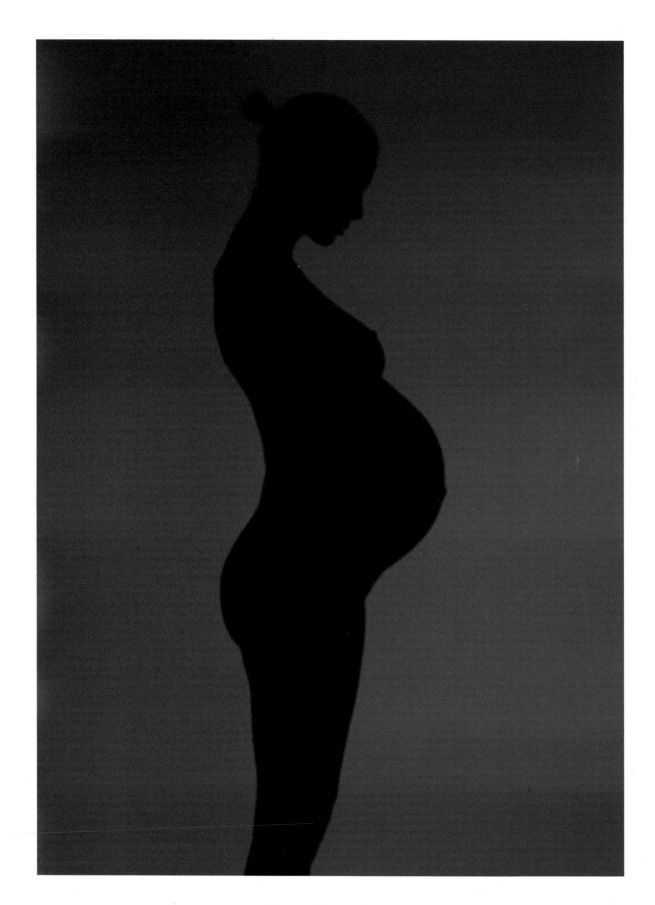

. . . and a new journey begins . . .

# photography credits *(The following photos were used by permission.)*

## I want to thank all of the photographers for the use of their photos in my book!

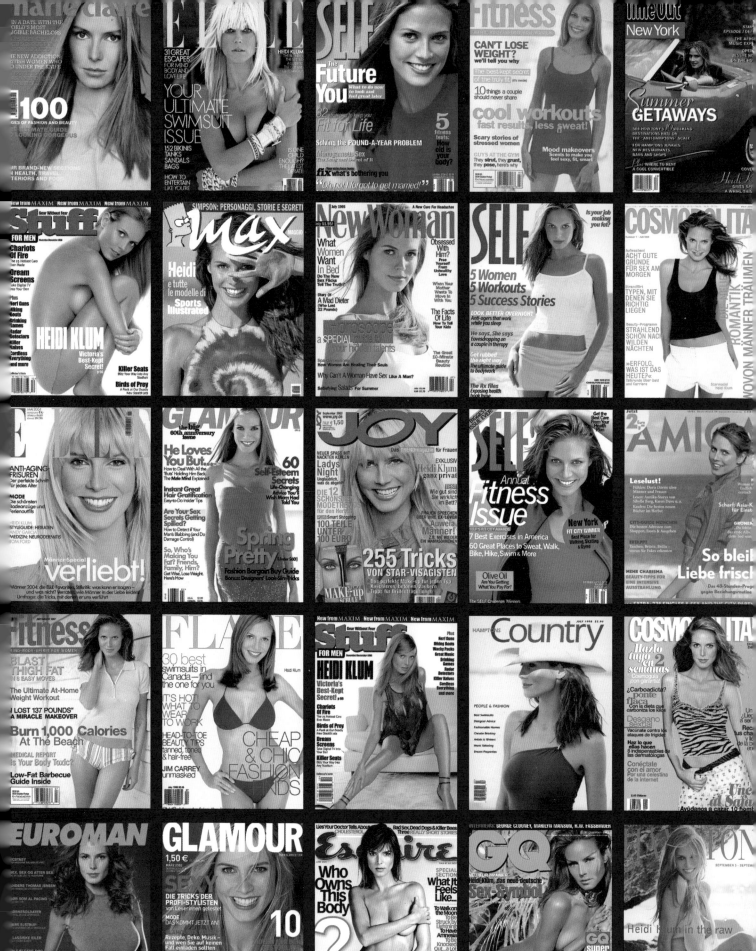